Discriminative Stimulus Properties of Drugs

ADVANCES IN BEHAVIORAL BIOLOGY

Editorial Board:

Jan Bures	Institute of Physiology, Prague, Czechoslovakia
Irwin Kopin	National Institute of Mental Health, Bethesda, Maryland
Bruce McEwen	Rockefeller University, New York, New York
James McGaugh	University of California, Irvine, California
Karl Pribram	Stanford University School of Medicine, Stanford, California
Jay Rosenblatt	Rutgers University, Newark, New Jersey
Lawrence Weiskrantz	University of Oxford, Oxford, England

Recent Volumes in this Series

Volume 10 • NEUROHUMORAL CODING OF BRAIN FUNCTION
  Edited by R. D. Myers and René Raúl Drucker-Colín • 1974

Volume 11 • REPRODUCTIVE BEHAVIOR
  Edited by William Montagna and William A. Sadler • 1974

Volume 12 • THE NEUROPSYCHOLOGY OF AGGRESSION
  Edited by Richard E. Whalen • 1974

Volume 13 • ANEURAL ORGANISMS IN NEUROBIOLOGY
  Edited by Edward M. Eisenstein • 1975

Volume 14 • NUTRITION AND MENTAL FUNCTIONS
  Edited by George Serban • 1975

Volume 15 • SENSORY PHYSIOLOGY AND BEHAVIOR
  Edited by Rachel Galun, Peter Hillman, Itzhak Parnas,
  and Robert Werman • 1975

Volume 16 • NEUROBIOLOGY OF AGING
  Edited by J. M. Ordy and K. R. Brizzee • 1975

Volume 17 • ENVIRONMENTS AS THERAPY FOR BRAIN DYSFUNCTION
  Edited by Roger N. Walsh and William T. Greenough • 1976

Volume 18 • NEURAL CONTROL OF LOCOMOTION
  Edited by Richard M. Herman, Sten Grillner, Paul S. G. Stein,
  and Douglas G. Stuart • 1976

Volume 19 • THE BIOLOGY OF THE SCHIZOPHRENIC PROCESS
  Edited by Stewart Wolf and Beatrice Bishop Berle • 1976

Volume 20 • THE SEPTAL NUCLEI
  Edited by Jon F. DeFrance • 1976

Volume 21 • COCAINE AND OTHER STIMULANTS
  Edited by Everett H. Ellinwood, Jr. and M. Marlyne Kilbey • 1977

Volume 22 • DISCRIMINATIVE STIMULUS PROPERTIES OF DRUGS
  Edited by Harbans Lal • 1977

A Continuation Order Plan is available for this series. A continuation order will bring delivery of each new volume immediately upon publication. Volumes are billed only upon actual shipment. For further information please contact the publisher.

Discriminative Stimulus Properties of Drugs

Edited by

Harbans Lal
University of Rhode Island, Kingston

PLENUM PRESS · NEW YORK AND LONDON

Library of Congress Cataloging in Publication Data

Main entry under title:

Discriminative stimulus properties of drugs.

(Advances in behavioral biology; v. 22)
Includes index.
1. Psychopharmacology. 2. Drugs—Physiological effect. 3. Drugs—Psychological aspects. I. Harbans Lal. [DNLM: 1. Drugs. QV38 D449]
RM315.D58   615'.78   77-1805
ISBN 0-306-37922-8

© 1977 Plenum Press, New York
A Division of Plenum Publishing Corporation
227 West 17th Street, New York, N.Y. 10011

All rights reserved

No part of this book may be reproduced, stored in a retrieval system, or transmitted, in any form or by any means, electronic, mechanical, photocopying, microfilming, recording, or otherwise, without written permission from the Publisher

Printed in the United States of America

Foreword

As one who has gone down the wayward path from "pure" organic chemistry to biochemistry to pharmacology, I was not quite prepared to go all the way - into the field of discriminable stimuli. The organizer of the symposium on discriminable stimuli induced by drugs, Dr. Harbans Lal, did seduce me into attending. Having lost my behavioral virginity, I now stare with open eyes at the field. One item in particular at this meeting exemplifies to me the power of such techniques. Dr. Albert Weissman mentioned the problem he tackled with getting rats to discriminate between saline and dilute solutions of aspirin. Under ordinary circumstances, the animals could not perform this task. However, if the animals were sensitized by injection of prostaglandin into their foot pads, then they were capable of discriminating even very dilute solutions of aspirin. In a sense, Al had created a model of the human arthritic who can jolly well tell if you have given him an aspirin or a salt tablet.

The reader of this volume will find it a good introduction to the utilization of discriminable stimuli induced by drugs. After a preface by the organizer, two experts discuss basic principles in separate chapters. One of these chapters places emphasis on the drugs; the other places emphasis on the induced cues and states. As a concluding chapter, there is a summary of past research in the field as well as speculation on the future. These speculations have value since they are made by one of the long-term workers in the field: Dr. Lal.

Between the introduction and the summary, there are chapters on a number of classes of psychotropic drugs which have been studied with regard to discriminable stimuli: narcotic analgesics, narcotic antagonists, marihuana, alcohol and other CNS depressants, nicotinic drugs, hallucinogens, psychomotor stimulants, benzodiazepines. Clearly the emphasis is more on abused drugs than on psychotherapeutic drugs, but my prediction is that the technique will be applied increasingly to the study of psychotherapeutic drugs. This latter application may require the preconditioning of animals (similar to that in the aspirin study).

In one chapter, that of Altman et al., there is a summary of human studies using drugs as discriminative events. Undoubtedly such human studies will also be an area of increasing importance in the near future. This chapter and its excellent bibliography should serve as a good base for clinical applications.

All in all, I found the meeting fascinating and useful and I would not be surprised if many a reader found this volume similarly fascinating and useful.

                                            Earl Usdin, Ph.D.
                                            Chief
                                            Pharmacology Section
                                            National Institute of Mental Health

Preface

Availability of drugs has long been a bonanza to researchers in many fields. But in the field of behavioral biology and behavioral medicine it has played a particularly critical role. With drugs, researchers have been able to tease out behavioral processes and disease states for understanding their mechanisms which have otherwise defied investigation. The biochemical changes that drugs produce in the brain and the changes which are then reflected in neurophysiology and in altered states of behavior are measured quite reliably as unconditional and conditional responses. This chain of events specifically induced by drugs provides a unique system for scientific study of interdependent biological processes. Drug effects are readily reversible and can be replicated with reliability.

Drugs can be considered as a class of stimuli with properties so complex and varied that conventional stimuli such as light and sound, no matter how complex, seem to be barren by comparison. Drugs provide stimuli of many kinds. Their acute actions are often considered as unconditional stimuli. Some drugs serve as positive or negative reinforcers. Recently, a few drugs have been found to serve as conditional stimuli, a finding which has greatly facilitated understanding of placebo effects.

The present book extensively reviews a newly recognized function of drugs; namely their ability to act as discriminative stimuli. When a pharmacological action is psychologically perceived a drug is said to have formed a discriminative stimulus. In this case the focus is not on what the drug does to the subject, but rather on how the subject's behavior reflects his realization that drug is acting in his body. What is innovative in this is that, whereas in the past discrimination studies have always utilized externally presented physical events as stimuli, now the changes in the internal state of the subject become the focus of discrimination studies. This discovery led a number of researchers to design experiments in which they ask questions such as "Which drugs can and which cannot produce a discriminative stimulus?" and "When a drug is established as a discriminative stimulus, which drugs or physiological manipulations do and which do not generalize to this stimulus?" These questions are researched because they have implications in both basic and applied fields. Which effects of drugs provide the basis for drug discrimination? Can a peripherally acting effect of a drug be discriminated? Can stimulation or lesioning of selected brain areas generalize to or antagonize the drug stimuli? What are the rules under which drug discrimination is acquired or extinguished? Are drug stimuli related to the therapeutic effects?

There are many applied implications of drug-induced discriminable stimuli just as there are basic implications. Drug discrimination is already being looked into for its potential in providing a tool for the study of interoceptive stimuli, for study of chemical bases of euphoria, to develop animal models of disease states, to investigate biochemistry of mood alteration, and to establish new ways of predicting therapeutic as well as toxic effects of newly synthesized chemicals. Already drug discrimination data are being routinely utilized in decision making at early stages of drug development.

All of the above questions are reviewed for the first time in one volume by scientists who themselves pioneered research in this area. In addition, material compiled by one scientist is strengthened and modified by feedback from other scientists. Before each chapter of this book was completed, all of the authors were invited for a weekend retreat in New Hampshire to review together the contents of various chapters. Through this process ideas and suggestions generated out of collective thinking were incorporated in the final version of the manuscripts.

A glance over the contents of this book will reveal that the subject of drug discrimination has been treated rather extensively by the leaders in the field. Individual chapters examined discriminative stimuli formed by different classes of drugs. They also examine theoretical aspects of this newly emerging field of scientific inquiry. Applications of drug discrimination in broad areas of physiology, psychology, psychiatry, pharmacology, neurochemistry and medicine are discussed throughout the book. New approaches to drug development and animal models of human diseases are elaborated.

Psychologists, psychiatrists, pharmacologists and physiologists, whether in research or teaching, will find this book valuable. Also, graduate students in behavioral and medical sciences can benefit. This book will serve as a ready reference for pharmacologists, toxicologists, and chemists in pharmaceutical industry.

PREFACE

They can refer to this book for details of methodology and already available information applicable in drug development as all of the chapters are replete with actual data and illustrations. Because of the rapid publication of the book, the material is fresh and updated. The book was prepared with these objectives in mind. If these goals are accomplished I feel highly compensated for my efforts in putting this book together.

January 28, 1977   Harbans Lal

Acknowledgments

I wish to express my sincere gratitude and appreciation to the many friends and coworkers who have given of their time, effort and encouragement in the preparation of this volume. Many others interacted in numerous ways in perceiving and organizing concepts which are elaborated in this book. Even though it is impossible to acknowledge all of those who have contributed, I do wish to cite the folowing people for their support.

Dr. Paul Janssen made his laboratories available and Dr. Carlos Niemegeers and Mr. Francis Colpaert were team-mates in generating many data and concepts included in this book. Dr. Stuart Feilding, Dr. William J. Novik, Dr. David Tedeschi, and Dr. Albert Weissman provided encouragement and assistance in obtaining funds. Mary Alyce Conrad, Lucie A. Johnson and Kathleen McGovern carefully typed portions of the manuscript. Secretarial services were amply provided by Elda G. Pellerin. Dr. Gerald Gianutsos and Dr. Nelson Smith assisted in editorial work and Stephen Miksic proofread the material. Robert Gianforcaro, Gary Shearman and Stephen Miksic prepared the subject index. Lederle Laboratories, Hoescht-Roussell Pharmaceutical Inc., Pfizer, Inc., and Coulbourn Instrument Co. provided financial support. The staff of New England Center for Continuing Education provided excellent services during the meeting of contributors to finalize the material included in this manuscript. Dr. Earl Usdin of the National Institute of Mental Health was instrumental in arranging the publication of the abstracts in Psychopharmacological Communications.

I especially thank the contributors without whose timely support and excellent coverage of the material this boook could have never been completed. Appreciation is also due to the many investigators and publishers who generously gave permission to the authors to reproduce parts of their material.

Finally, a special acknowledgement is given to Plenum Press and its staff for their patience and helpful collaboration.

Contents

Drugs as Discriminative Stimuli 1
    Albert Weissman

Drug-Induced Cues and States: Some
Theoretical and Methodological Inferences 5
    Francis C. Colpaert

Discriminable Stimuli Produced by
Narcotic Analgesics 23
    Harbans Lal, Gerald Gianutsos,
    and Stephen Miksic

Discriminative Properties of Narcotic
Antagonists 47
    Stephen G. Holtzman, Harlan E. Shannon,
    and Gerald J. Schaefer

Discriminable Stimuli Produced by Alcohol
and Other CNS Depressants 73
    Herbert Barry III and Edward C. Krimmer

Discriminative Stimulus Properties of
Benzodiazepine and Barbiturates 93
    Francis C. Colpaert

Characterization of Discriminative Response
Control by Psychomotor Stimulants 107
    Peter B. Silverman and Beng T. Ho

Discriminable Stimuli Produced by
Marihuana Constituents 121
    Edward C. Krimmer and Herbert Barry III

Discriminative Stimulus Properties of
Hallucinogens: Behavioral Assay of
Drug Action 137
    Donald M. Kuhn, Francis J. White,
    and James B. Appel

Cholinergic and Non-Cholinergic Aspects of
the Discriminative Stimulus Properties of
Nicotine 155
    John A. Rosecrans and William T. Chance

Drugs as Discriminable Events in Humans 187
    Jack L. Altman, Jean-Marie Albert,
    Stephen L. Milstein, and Isaac Greenberg

Drug-Induced Discriminable Stimuli:
Past Research and Future Perspectives 207
    Harbans Lal

Index 233

DRUGS AS DISCRIMINATIVE STIMULI

Albert Weissman

Department of Pharmacology
Pfizer, Inc.
Groton, Conn. 06340

Drug studies have long been a magnet for behavioral biologists. The biochemical changes drugs produce in brain, the neurophysiological effects they bring about, their alterations of unconditioned and conditioned behavior, their interactions with stimuli-including drug stimuli-that produce all manner of central effects: all these subjects have been of utmost importance. Drugs may be considered as a class of stimuli with effects so varied that the usual stimuli that psychologists use as independent variables - lights, sounds, feeds, electric shocks -- seem barren by comparison.

The vast preponderance of drug studies focuses on unconditioned effects of drugs such as those classified above, that is, what drugs do to the subject when the experimenter administers them. This stimulus function of drugs is that of the unconditioned stimulus, and just as the sensory psychologist may be interested in absolute thresholds of unconditioned stimuli and behavioral differences in response to stimuli that vary along a single dimension, so the pharmacologist and psychopharmacologist may be interested in effective doses, dose-response curves and structure-activity relationships.

But experimental psychologists are particularly interested in examining functions of a stimulus other than its unconditioned effects. They want to know which stimuli may be conditioned in a Pavlovian paradigm and how. They want to know which stimuli can serve the functions of positive or negative reinforcers in operant experiments. And they want to know the mechanisms whereby a stimulus can set the occasion for a given response to be reinforced, that is, to become a discriminative stimulus.

Thus, there has been an explosion of work that focuses on the role of drugs as stimuli exerting functions other than those of unconditioned stimuli. Pavlovian experiments show that drugs can become conditioned stimuli; indeed this may be the best way of conceptualizing the mechanism of action of placeboes. A wealth of experimentation also shows that drugs may serve as reinforcing stimuli. Note that in such experiments the experimenter does not administer the drug to the subject: He only makes it available so that the subject can self-administer it. This field has enriched our conceptualization of drug abuse.

Work reported and reviewed in this volume surely comprises only the initial probes of an additional stimulus function that drugs can serve--that of a discriminative stimulus. In such experiments the focus is not on what the drug does to the animal, but rather on how the animal's behavior reflects his discrimination of the drug effect. For the most part, studies to date have addressed two kinds of questions: (1) which drugs can and which cannot be discriminated by animals, and (2) when a drug is established as a discriminative stimulus, which drugs do and which don't generalize to this stimulus. These subjects are no trivial exercise. They have important basic and applied implications. Can animals discriminate peripherally-acting drugs? After all, humans have no trouble telling when they have taken even an antibiotic, provided it causes a peripheral side effect such as diarrhea or an allergic response. Just what unconditioned effects provide the basis for drug discriminations? If an animal responds as if he discriminates an opiate, which of the many properties of the opiate serve as the cue? Generalization studies will, before long, give the answer. Not only may other drugs generalize to the drug cue, but so may electrical stimulation of selected brain areas, further enabling ultimate identification of the components of drug action responsible for discriminability.

In the practical sphere, drug discrimination studies will play an increasing role in decision making at early stages of drug discovery. Already, Janssen Laboratories have bolstered their claim that certain antidiarrheals derived structurally from narcotic type analgesics do not produce subjective effects in common with opiates, by using supportive drug discrimination studies in rodents. And already, fenfluramine has been shown not to generalize to its close analog, amphetamine, confirming clinical experience that fenfluramine, unlike many phenethylamine anorectics, does not produce the same subjective effects as amphetamine. It can be expected that the study of such "subjective effects" of drugs in animals will play an increasing preclinical role in facilitating prediction of abuse liability, although the inperfection of such procedures should not cause an overly sanguine view of their validity at this time.

Yet topics such as those mentioned above by no means exhaust the potential of this general area. The drug discrimination paradigm is only beginning to be exploited, and we can look forward to answers to questions such as these: Under what conditions can a subject discriminate what is usually a non-discriminable drug? If an animal exposed to a pathological condition is better able to discriminate a drug that is pallative, then new models of pathology can be tested in animals by such techniques. Can animals be taught to discriminate a single property common to several otherwise diverse drugs? Such generalization studies can yield information on the "analyzers" that are the basis of discrimination learning. What are the absolute drug dosage thresholds that can be discriminated? In the realm of sensory psychophysics, trained subjects can discriminate remarkably low intensities of sensory stimulation. Will animals be able to discriminate doses of centrally acting drugs that are lower than those that produce any unconditional effects? The scope of these and other conceivable drug discrimination investigations is extremely broad, because ultimately they encompass all the discrimination and generalization paradigms experimental psychologists have explored, but expanded with the richness of drug stimuli.

In this day of biochemical analysis of drug actions it is also a distinct pleasure to see a new behavioral area blossom that is not readily subject to reductionism. Biochemical tools offer little insight into why certain drugs selectively block conditioned avoidance behavior, reduce conditioned emotional reactions or alter self-stimulation response rates. They do not enable prediction of those agents that serve as reinforcers. And now drugs as cues! Experimental psychopharmacology at the conditioned behavioral level is alive and vibrant.

DRUG-PRODUCED CUES AND STATES: SOME THEORETICAL
AND METHODOLOGICAL INFERENCES

F.C. Colpaert

Dept. Pharmacology
Janssen Pharmaceutica Research Laboratories
B-2340 Beerse, Belgium

I. THE UNITARY CONCEPT

A major position in the field of Drug Discrimination (DD) and State-Dependent (StD) learning is that the learning phenomena referred to by these terms would pertain to a single property of drugs and require the operation of one type of physiological mechanisms. Acceptance of this concept is very widespread, and the following statements exemplify the position in a most explicit way: "Indeed, the whole field of studies under the heading 'state-dependent learning' seems to me to be no more and no less than examples of control of behavior by drugs as discriminative stimuli." (Dews, 1975); "... that state-dependent (i.e. discriminative stimulus) properties ... of drugs ..." (Kuhn et al., 1976).

The development and specification of this concept is largely based upon the outstanding and extensive work by Overton (e.g. 1964, 1966, 1968, 1971, 1974). Some major points characterizing the concept are: (1) DD and StD learning reflect the different procedures used but do not indicate that different properties of drugs might be responsible for the two effects; (2) drugs must act on the brain

in order to be able to give rise to such learning phenomena; (3) in
the context of stimulus control by drugs, the following terms are
essentially interchangeable: dissociation, state-dependency, discrimination; response transfer and stimulus generalization; state and
discriminative stimulus. Overton (1971) also argues against the
hypothesis that drugs may control responding by inducing distinctive
sensory cues that acquire response control through the operation of
sensory discrimination learning.

II. THE DUAL CONCEPT

Quite opposite to the former concept is another one (Colpaert et al., 1976a) holding that DD and StD learning represent
distinct and essentially unrelated phenomena. Some of its basic
assumptions are: (1) there are two distinct types of stimulus control
by drugs. One is instrumental in DD learning; it requires the drug
to produce a perceivable change in the organism's internal environment. This perceivable change constitutes a stimulus which, in
addition, must be discriminable from solvent injection. The drug
versus solvent injection should then be applied as a discriminandum
in an otherwise ordinary discrimination task. The second type is
denoted as StD learning; in this case, the drug is one of the stimuli
constituting the entire set of the internal and external conditions
which prevail during the establishment of a predetermined (classical
or operant) learning process. It may appear that what is acquired
under this set of conditions, does not transfer to the same set when
the drug is omitted; in this case, the learning effect is said to be
conditional ("dependent") upon drug administration (or the "state" thus
induced); (2) the learning mechanisms involved in these two types of
stimulus control are not identical, and the stimulus function of a
drug in DD learning is distinct from that in StD learning; (3) the pharmacological properties which are responsible for a drug's ability to
produce an effective discriminative stimulus, are not necessarily
similar to those which underlie its possible capacity to produce a
state upon which learning effects can be made conditional; (4) a drug-
produced discriminative stimulus should be termed a Discriminative
Stimulus Complex (DSC). This notion accounts for the possibility
that the stimulus thus defined may be composed of pharmacologically
and/or functionally heterogenous components which may differ considerably as regards their relevance to the composed entity, or complex; (5) DD learning, unlike StD learning, does not require the drug
to act centrally. This assumption holds that any perceivable drug-
produced change (whether relevant or not) in either the CNS or the
periphery can potentially act as a discriminative stimulus. Whether
it will acutally do so depends primarily on the relative strength and
distinctiveness of the change.
It should be noted that assumptions 2 to 4 are extensions of the first
one, and that the central position concerns the distinction itself between DD and StD learning.

III. DRUG-PRODUCED CUES AND STATES

To show that DD learning is something different from StD learning requires evidence indicating that a drug can produce a cue on the one hand, and a state upon which learning effects can be made conditional on the other. It would be still more conclusive (and convincing, perhaps) to reveal that the cue and the state typically produced by a single class of drugs, are characterized distinctly along some relevant pharmacological, biochemical or physiological parameters.

We are now able to present such evidence; the most pertinent data pertain to narcotic analgesic drugs, and the available literature on the stimulus properties of these drugs has been reviewed very recently (Colpaert, 1976). In the present volume, the topic has already been discussed by Lal and Holtzman, and it may be sufficient, therefore, to mention here only some of the conclusions reached in our review: (1) narcotic analgesics possess discriminative stimulus properties (narcotic cue), and are able to produce a state upon which responses (or learning effects in general) can be made conditional (narcotic state); (2) 5-hydroxytryptamine is critically involved in the narcotic state, but not in the narcotic cue; (3) the narcotic state, unlike the narcotic cue, is subject to tolerance. The major evidence substantiating the second and the third conclusion can be summarized as follows: Rosecrans and his collaborators found that the ability of narcotics to control operant responding decreased from 100 % to 0 % following a single p-chlorophenylalanine (p-CPA) administration (Rosecrans et al., 1973), and that this ability was subject to tolerance (Hirschhorn and Rosecrans, 1974). In contrast, we found that the cuing properties of narcotics are not affected by the same p-CPA administration, nor by other treatments presumably decreasing or increasing central serotonergic activity (Colpaert et al., 1976g). We have also been able to show that tolerance to these cuing effects does not develop over a period as long as 4 months after training (Colpaert et al., 1976b).
The least one can conclude from these seemingly conflicting findings is, that Rosecrans's laboratory and ours have been studying phenomena which differ quite dramatically in some pharmacological and physiological respects. It can be inferred, from this, that narcotic analgesics may control operant behavior in two different ways, and that the stimulus properties involved in these two types of response control are distinct (Colpaert, 1976). This implies that it does not make much sense to use the term "the stimulus properties of drugs" if it is meant to represent a unitary drug property and to refer to a single physiological process (quite apart from the fact that the term should include mere unconditioned in addition to still other stimulus properties of drugs as well).
A further inference (Colpaert, 1976) is that the phenomenon we have been investigating (Colpaert et al., 1976b, 1976g) should be identified as the discriminative stimulus properties of narcotic analgesics, whereas those studied in the two other reports (Rosecrans et al.,

1973; Hirschhorn and Rosecrans, 1974) represent StD learning effects.

The treatment of the narcotic cue and the narcotic state as special cases of DD and StD learning respectively (Colpaert, 1976), allows to accept the first three of the abovementioned assumptions characterizing the dual concept.
The fourth assumption, i.e. the one about the complex composition of the cuing properties of drugs, has been substantiated by the demonstration (Colpaert et al., 1976e) of asymmetrical generalization between the narcotic analgesic fentanyl (Janssen et al., 1963) and the dopamine receptor agonist, apomorphine (Colpaert et al., 1976h). These two drugs possess intrinsic discriminative stimulus properties (Colpaert et al., 1975a, 1975b), and it was found (Colpaert et al., 1976e) that apomorphine is not generalized with fentanyl in rats trained to discriminate fentanyl from saline, but that fentanyl does produce the apomorphine-DSC in rats trained to discriminate the latter from saline. This and other data (Colpaert et al., 1976e) indicate that part of the narcotic cue is constituted by an apomorphine-like stimulus, and that the latter constitutes one out of the probably several components composing the narcotic DSC.
The fifth assumption holds that DD learning, unlike StD learning, does not require the drug to act on the brain. That the phenomenon of state-dependency is of a central nature may be true in as much as states are centrally processed events. Whether a drug must exert a central action to produce such a state, is less certain; it is conceivable that the massive impact which some compounds (e.g. noradrenaline) have at peripheral sites, may indirectly "bring" the organism into a state upon which learning effects may be made conditional. Regardless of the latter speculation, however, the general consensus is that drugs should act centrally in order to induce state-dependency, and the point to be made here is, that this does not apply to DD learning. Thus, data have been presented (Colpaert et al., 1975c) which show that a peripheral anticholinergic, isopropamide, does produce a DSC, and that stimulus generalization with this DSC is based upon peripheral anticholinergic activity. It is interesting to note, at this point, that the DSC produced by low dl-amphetamine doses, unlike the state (Roffman and Lal, 1972) or the DSC (Schechter and Rosecrans, 1973) produced by high doses of the same drug, is probably of peripheral origin (Colpaert et al., 1976f). This exemplifies the fact that there may exist qualitative in addition to quantitative differences between the stimulus properties of the same drug at different dose levels.

IV. METHODOLOGICAL PROBLEMS

The distinction between the physiological processes governing drug-produced cues and states necessitates the development of specific methods allowing to investigate these two phenomena in their own right. Overton (1974) has offered a number of excellent recommendations for StD learning methods, and their strict observance will undoubtedly result in very satisfactory data. Apart from some rather general considerations (Colpaert et al., 1976a), the methodology of DD learning has been somewhat neglected. A large variety of methods and procedures are currently used by different investigators. This may be beneficial to the extent that different approaches lead to equivocal results; in this case, the general nature of the finding over various procedural variables may increase the relevance of the conclusion derived from it. The use of different procedures is also of interest when the intention is to investigate the significance of the procedural variables themselves. However, the situation becomes more dubious when procedures appear to lead readily to incorrect interpretations, as will be discussed below.

Another complicating circumstance is, that different procedures may define the cuing properties of drugs at different levels of specificity; in a recent study (Colpaert et al., 1976d) on the cuing properties of the benzodiazepines and related drugs, it was found that the DSC produced by these drugs constitute a pharmacologically highly specific phenomenon. It was also shown that the neuroleptics haloperidol and chlorpromazine are not generalized with the benzodiazepine-DSC, and later experiments (unpublished data) revealed that this DSC is not antagonized by amphetamine. The above and other results have allowed us to conclude (Colpaert et al., 1976d) that the benzodiazepine-DSC is not subserved by the general depressant or sedative effects of these drugs. This is in direct contrast to the conclusion reached by other authors (Barry, 1974; Barry and Krimmer, 1975; Overton, 1966, 1971) who found that chlorpromazine is partially generalized with the benzodiazepine-DSC, and that amphetamine may partially antagonize this DSC. This apparent discrepancy can be effectively accounted for by assuming that, owing to differences in procedures, the cuing properties of the benzodiazepines or related drugs had been defined at different levels of specificity (for discussion see: Colpaert et al., 1976d). Defining the cuing properties of drugs at a low level of specificity is not itself incorrect, but is simply less interesting; clearly, having rats discriminating, say, between the mere presence or absence of drug – whatever the nature of the drug – is of no scientific interest. Having rats able to detect the injection of a narcotic, as opposed to any other drug-class, is exactly what DD learning should be about.

An adequate method for DD learning studies should incorporate the following two features: (1) the method should produce data pertaining exclusively to the cuing properties of drugs, without being confounded by irrelevant training- or drug effects; (2) it should define these properties at a high level of specificity, such that drug-class specific rather than more inclusive drug effects be measured. It would be fortunate, though not strictly necessary, if the method could also provide some indications of the behavioral toxicity of the drugs being studied. Such a method has been described elsewhere (Colpaert et al., 1976a), and there is abundant data (e.g. Colpaert et al., 1975a, 1976c, 1976d) demonstrating that this method matches the requirement outlined above. In the further discussion, we will try to explain how other more commonly employed methods may sometimes fail to do so.

1 - The Skinnerian method

Learning theorists in the field of discrimination learning have been much inspired by the Skinnerian method, and its use in the field of DD learning is a logical extension of a fruitful tradition. The method essentially consists of training an animal to respond in the presence of one stimulus (the go-stimulus; S^+) and not to respond in the presence of another one (the no-go-stimulus; S^-). After training, stimulus generalization tests assess the relative occurrence of the response in the presence of novel stimuli physically different from both S^+ and S^-. This measurement is assumed to be directly proportional to the degree of perceptual generalization of the test stimulus to S^+.

In his interesting work on the cuing properties of drugs, Winter (e.g. 1973, 1974) has adopted this method for the study of DD learning. Typically, two groups of animals are used. In one group (I) saline is the S^+, whereas the training drug constitutes the S^-; in the other group (II), the stimulus assignments are reversed. Our criticism of this method is two-fold. Firstly, training animals to emit a particular response while being drugged (as is the case for group II) may readily result in state-dependency of the learning effect. To the extent that the state-dependency may be symmetrical, the same may apply to group I, and the results produced may be at least partially loaded by StD learning effects (instead of, or in addition to, discriminative stimulus control). Although measures can be taken to avoid the occurrence of state-dependency (such as establishing the response before the introduction of the discriminandum; see Colpaert et al., 1976a), the actual presence of such effects should be assessed.
The second criticism relates to the susceptibility of this method to rate-modulating drug effects. A purely hypothetical case may exemplify this issue. Test drug γ is tested in two groups I and II trained to discriminate training drug X from saline as outlined above, and suppose that γ exerts marked rate-depressant effects. Hypothetical test data are given in Fig. 1. At least 2 assumptions can be made concerning the cuing properties of γ. <u>Assumption 1</u> is that γ does not produce an X-like DSC. In this case, responding in group I will be saline-like (high rate) because of lack of X-like cuing properties. At higher doses, response rate will decrease because of intrinsic rate-depressant effects of γ. In group II, responding will be saline-like (low rate) because of lack of X-like cuing properties, and because reponding will be depressed anyway. The slight and inconsistent increase at dose c of γ (Fig. 1) seems to be due to ordinary variability, and does not reach statistical significance ($p > .05$).
<u>Assumption 2</u> is that γ does produce an X-like DSC. In this case,

responding in group I will be relatively high at the doses a and b because the DSC is not yet apparent; at higher doses (c and d), responding will decrease because of increasing generalization with the X-DSC, and because responding is suppressed anyway. In group II, responding will be low (saline-like) at doses a and b because the DSC is not yet apparent. At higher doses (c and d) responding is subject to two mutually opposed tendencies; one is response increase because of progressive generalization of γ with X; the other is decrease because of increasingly severe rate-depressant effects of γ.

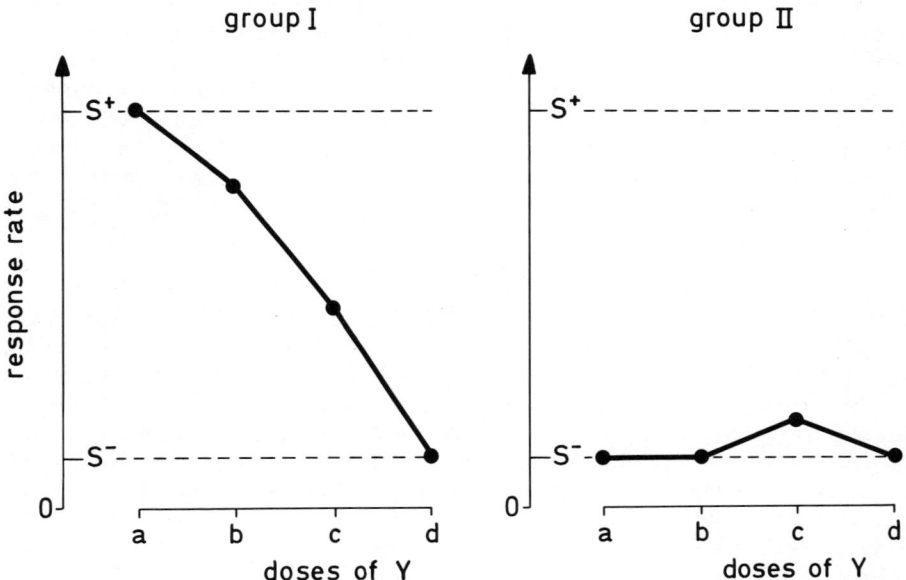

Fig. 1. Hypothetical test data on test drug γ from rats trained to discriminate X from saline according to the Skinnerian method.
The dashed lines indicate response levels after S^+ and S^-; S^+ and S^- are the go- and the no-go-stimulus respectively. S^+ = saline and S^- = X in group I; in group II, S^+ = X and S^- = saline. The solid lines represent test data with different doses (a to d) of γ.

The test curve for group II may assume an almost indefinite number of different shapes because the relative contribution by the two sources of variation (i.e. stimulus generalization and rate-depressant effects) may vary very much; (1) the slope of the positively accelerated part of the curve is determined by the cuing properties of γ; (2) the slope of the negatively accelerated part of the curve is determined by the rate-depressant effect of γ; (3) the amplitude of the curve depends upon the values of (1) and (2) at any point of the

dose-axis.
As the slopes and the doses for cuing are not covariant with those for rate-depressant effects of drugs (Colpaert et al., 1975a, 1976b, 1976d; a rule which, interestingly, may not apply to state-dependency, see: Grilly, 1975) it will be extremely difficult to determine the contribution of the cuing effects to the results obtained. The situation gets even more complex when the drugs being studied may increase as well as decrease responding and when inter- and intraindividual variability at different doses is very high (as is the case for benzodiazepines, see: Colpaert et al., 1976d). To cope with these difficulties, numerous and elaborate control groups would be required and, indeed, a general solution is not at hand (Winter, 1975). As a result, the test data (Fig. 1) discussed here can be predicted on the basis of two entirely opposite assumptions regarding the cuing properties of the drug tested. It is interesting to note that actual test data very similar to those depicted in Fig. 1 have made Winter (1974) conclude that 3,4-dimethoxyphenylethylamine does not produce the mescaline-DSC <u>even at rate-depressant doses</u>. This may be true, but it appears that such a conclusion can not be justified by the type of data discussed here.

2 - Superimposition

The most widely used method in the field of DD learning consists of superimposing the training procedures for groups I and II of the Skinnerian method, in a single group of animals. Thus, rats are trained to execute one response (R_1) upon injection with the training drug (S_1), and to execute another one (R_2) upon saline (S_2) injection. R_2 is ineffective after S_1 and R_1 is ineffective after S_2. Again, the possible occurrence of state-dependency can be avoided by establishing R_1 and R_2 before discrimination training is started. In any case, possible StD learning effects can be readily detected as is shown below.

The criticism here concerns the measurement of discriminative responding. That is, a percentage of drug-correct responses (% d-c R), typically assessed in the course of an extinction trial, is commonly employed as an index of stimulus generalization. The data are evaluated against performance under training conditions S_1 and S_2, and this performance usually varies between 70 and 90 % d-c R under training drug, and between 10 and 30 % d-c R under saline. There are several points which merit attention here. The first one is that, in discrimination learning, a relatively low level (such as 70 % to 90 % d-c R) of training criterion results in overinclusive stimulus generalization (e.g. Doty and Rutledge, 1959). The second point is, that the assessment of % d-c R during an extinction trial yields typically flat stimulus generalization gradients (Rilling <u>et al.</u> 1975), thus indicating that the dimension along which stimulus generalization is assessed, is relatively unspecific. An extinction trial also sets the opportunity for response probing to occur; the confounding influence of this effect is particularly severe with positive rein-

forcement (see below). In addition, extinction trials tend to wash
out the effects of training since the response contingencies are not
the same in testing as in training (Woodard and Bitterman, 1974).
Finally, discriminative stimuli may readily exert control over which
of two responses is to be executed, but not over response rate
(Migler and Millenson, 1969). These and other (Heise, 1975; Ray
and Sidman, 1970) arguments indicate that response rate, or any
measurement derived therefrom, has limited relevance to the stimulus generalization being studied.

Thus, the use of % d-c R as an index for stimulus generalization suffers from overinclusiveness and relative lack of specificity,
and may readily lead to erroneous and/or discordant interpretations.
A prototype of results yielding discordant interpretations is 50 %
d-c R after a given test treatment. Perusal of the literature reveals
that such a result is interpreted in three different ways. One is that
50 % differs from the saline control level (10-30 %) and hence corresponds best to the training drug condition; it may then be concluded
that the test drug was generalized with the training drug. Another
is that 50 % differs from the training drug control level (70-90 %)
and hence corresponds best to the saline condition; it may then be
concluded that the test drug was generalized with the training drug.
A third interpretation is that 50 % d-c R corresponds to neither the
training drug nor the saline condition; it may be inferred that the test
result differs qualitatively from either training condition, and that
50 % is a chance level. The latter interpretation is entirely inappropriate for two reasons; (1) there is no such thing as chance performance in animals which are trained to discriminate perfectly between
two stimuli; (2) the interpretation that 50 % denotes a qualitative difference between the test drug and both training conditions, is not
maintained when the 50 % result is part of a dose-response curve
running from 20 % ($\pm$ 10) to 80 % ($\pm$ 10); in the latter case, the 50 %
point would be said to indicate that, at this dose-level, the test drug
differs only quantitatively, but not qualitatively, from the training
drug. In other words, 50 % d-c R may be interpreted as an indication for either a qualitative difference from both training treatments,
or a mere quantitative difference between test- and training drug,
and there seems to be no way of avoiding this ambiguity.

3 - Response selection versus percentage of drug-correct responses

To cope with the difficulties inherent in the superimposition method, we have introduced a "response selection" procedure
(Colpaert et al., 1975a, 1976a). The method and all its procedural
features have been described in much detail elsewhere (Colpaert et
al., 1976a), and a fair amount of data thus obtained has been reported (e.g. Colpaert et al., 1976c, 1976d).

We will now present some direct evidence indicating the
superiority of the "response selection" procedure over the "% d-c R"

procedure.

By response selection is meant here that the animals are required to select either of two levers in a food-reinforced two-lever operant situation. Lever selection is measured as that lever upon which a total of 10 responses is made first by rats trained to press (FR 10) one lever (Drug Lever: DL) after training drug treatment, and another one (Saline Lever: SL) after saline.

It will be shown that even in rats thus trained, and which typically reach a 100 % correct level of performance, the use of "% d-c R" in an extinction trial results in a poor and inadequate measurement of discrimination. <u>Experiment 1</u>: Rats (n=6) were trained to discriminate 0.04 mg/kg fentanyl (s.c., t-30') from saline (s.c., t-30'); data on training and subsequent performance were similar to those previously reported (e.g. Colpaert <u>et al.</u>, 1975a) for rats trained according to this method. Upon presentation of either training stimulus (0.04 mg/kg fentanyl or saline), all six animals always selected the appropriate lever, and further responding was likewise at the 100 %-correct level. Test sessions were held under the following four conditions: (1) extinction (no reinforcement) session preceded by 0.04 mg/kg fentanyl; (2) extinction session preceded by saline; (3) a session during which pressing the incorrect lever (i.e. SL) was reinforced following 0.04 mg/kg fentanyl, and (4) a session during which pressing the incorrect lever (i.e. DL) was reinforced following saline. The sequence of test conditions was randomized, and the selected lever, and total responses were recorded. The results are represented in Fig. 2; it is shown that lack of reinforcement (conditions 1 and 2) generates response probing, thus resulting in an inferior % d-c R. It is evident that the drop in % d-c R from 100 % to $\pm$ 80 % is not due to a sudden loss of discrimination, and that this percentage is a poor and inaccurate measurement of the ability of these animals to discriminate fentanyl from saline. Indeed, each rat selected the treatment-appropriate lever upon either treatment, and the lever selection measurement appears to provide an entirely adequate index of discrimination. The results under conditions 3 and 4 demonstrate two major characteristics of responding in these rats. One is that this responding is not state-dependent because the animals are able to press the inappropriate lever at a rate equal to or sometimes higher than that observed under the corresponding training treatment. The second characteristic is, that whereas lever selection itself is under the discriminative control of the preceding drug- or saline injection, subsequent responding is certainly not. In fact, the distribution of subsequent responding over the two levers appears to be determined primarily by the reinforcement contingency applied. Hence, the % d-c R is primarily under the discriminative control of reinforcement and only to a minor extent of the stimulus presented before the session. That this percentage is better under no-reinforcement (conditions 1 and 2) as compared to incorrect reinforcement (conditions 3 and 4) indicates that the animals "expect" to obtain food by pressing the treatment-appropriate lever. However, the non-consolidation of this expectation appears to produce less predictable responding (compare conditions 1 and 2 with control, and

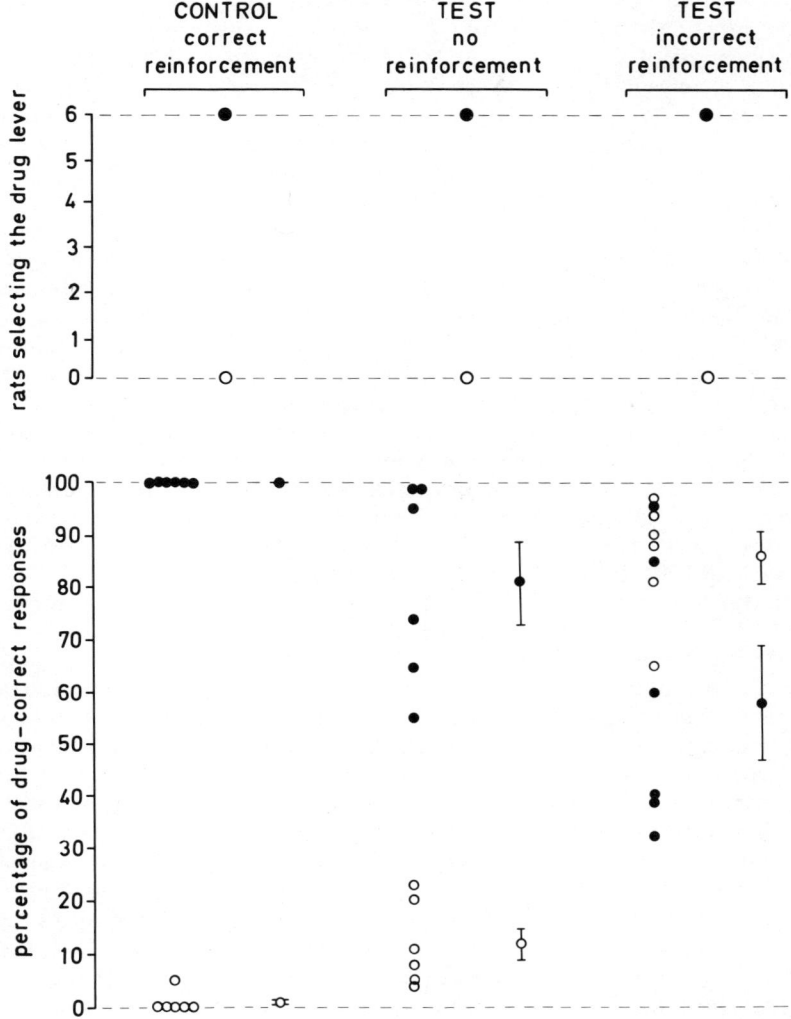

Fig. 2. Influence of no reinforcement and of incorrect reinforcement on two indices of discrimination in rats trained to discriminate 0.04 mg/kg fentanyl from saline.
Data were obtained during sessions preceded by either 0.04 mg/kg fentanyl (●) or saline (o). Individual data as well as group means ($\pm$ 1 SEM) are represented.

conditions 3 and 4 with 1 and 2), and this in turn explains the high variability typically observed with such data. An interesting though not really surprising observation is that, under incorrect reinforcement, treatment-appropriate lever pressing was somewhat better following fentanyl than following saline. This may suggest that the actual presence of a stimulus (i.e. the continuing fentanyl action) exerts more powerful discriminative control over responding than its absence does. The possibility of asymmetrical state-dependency can not account for this phenomenon because the rate at which incorrect responses were executed (on a min basis) would regularly exceed the control rate. The susceptibility of the % d-c R measurement to variables concerned with reinforcement also predicts that extinction will have a smaller impact on the variability of negatively reinforced (avoidance) as compared to that of positively reinforced responding. This is because the omission of reward following an otherwise positively reinforced response is noticed more rapidly than the omission of punishment which otherwise would also have been avoided. Thus, given the intensity of reinforcement being equal, extinction will proceed more slowly with negative reinforcement than with positive reinforcement, and the deleterious effects of extinction on the % d-c R measurement will be less marked with negative reinforcement.

Experiment 2: The second experiment was done in another group (n=6) of similarly trained rats. These animals received three fentanyl injections (0.01, 0.02 and 0.04 mg/kg); they then were allowed to select the lever of their choice, but once lever selection had been established, further responding on the selected lever was either reinforced (condition 1) or not (condition 2). It appeared (Fig. 3) that the measurement of lever selection provided an unequivocal index of stimulus generalization. Lever selection data were identical under both conditions, and this demonstrates the high reproducibility of the results thus established. It appeared again that the % d-c R measurement is less accurate, less predictable, and that it may lead to incorrect interpretations. Thus, the mean percentage was 66 % following 0.02 mg/kg fentanyl under condition 1; this result could be interpreted as evidence for "some generalization". The lever selection data, in contrast, indicate that there was no such thing as "some generalization", but that 4 animals showed generalization, whereas 2 did not. When no reinforcement was given (condition 2), the line connecting the mean % d-c R was somewhat flattened as compared with condition 1. Since control data in this group of animals were typically at the 100 %-correct level, it can easily be shown that the % d-c R following all three test treatments was significantly different from both training stimulus levels. It is obvious that straightforward conclusions cannot be drawn from these data.

The 55 % d-c R following 0.02 mg/kg fentanyl under condition 2 is a classical case of "intermediate" responding, or of responding at the "chance level". According to the lever selection data, however, it appeared that 4 out of 6 rats generalized this dose with the training dose; after having made 50 responses on the drug lever, one of them turned to the saline lever and made over 100 responses on it. The other 5 animals responded predominantly on either the drug- or the saline lever.

From the experiments described above, it follows that there

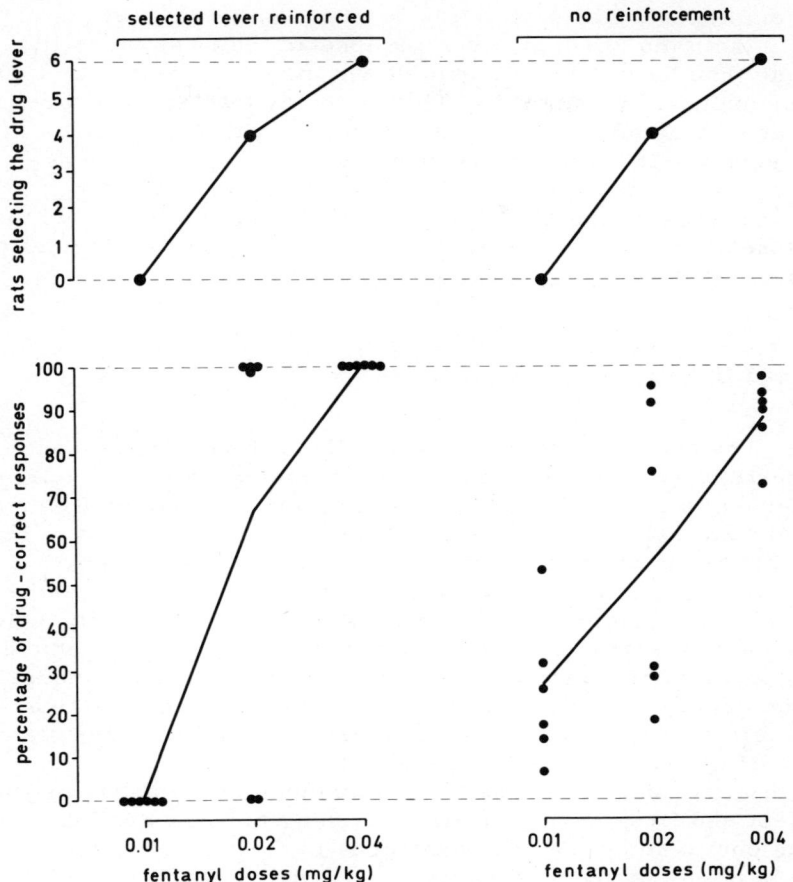

Fig. 3. Influence of reinforcement versus no reinforcement on two indices of generalization following different fentanyl doses. In the lower part of the graph, the points represent individual data; the lines connect group means.

is no reason to use % d-c R as a measurement of stimulus generalization, given the fact that a much superior index (i.e. lever selection or, in general, response selection) is available. The former measurement, as compared with the latter, is less accurate, less straightforward, and is much more susceptible to numerous variables (such as reinforcement, response bias, response probing, frustration effects) which produce a considerable amount of irrelevant variability.

There is also a theoretical rationale to the use of response selection rather than % d-c R as a measurement of stimulus generalization. That is, a drug-produced DSC should be conceived (Colpaert et al., 1976a) as a unique complex which, as such, bears little similarity to other complexes. The problem to be submitted to the laboratory animal is not: "do you find (, say,) amphetamine to be more like morphine than like saline?", but "do you find this drug to be typically morphine-like or not?". This is to say that the measurement should be of a nominal nature, because that is the very nature of the phenomenon itself. That the response selection procedure does produce highly specific data is indicated by data (Colpaert et al., 1976c, 1976d) showing that the cuing properties of drugs thus defined may very closely correlate with other most typical pharmacological properties of the same drugs.

V. CONCLUSION

The above comments on some theoretical and methodological aspects of research in the field of "stimulus control" by drugs are intended to emphasize, first and foremost, that Drug Discrimination and State-Dependent learning are distinct phenomena. This distinction has numerous consequences at all levels of study. Thus, the stimulus function is different in the two cases, and the same applies to the physiological processes involved. The pharmacological actions which are responsible for the cuing properties of some drugs do no appear to be identical to those underlying the state induced by the same drugs, and this point is heavily documented by a clear-cut case of differential features characterizing the DSC and the state of a single drug-class (Colpaert, 1976).
Differential recommendations for the methods in the areas of State-Dependent and Drug Discrimination learning are now available, thus enabling one to study the two phenomena in their own right. The emphasis is on the "purity" as well as on the "specificity" of the data produced by different methods, and observance of the basic principles outlined here and elsewhere (Overton, 1974, Colpaert et al., 1976a) may reduce the occurrence of confusing data and erroneous interpretations.

VI. REFERENCES

BARRY III, H.: Classification of drugs according to their discriminable effects in rats. Fed.Proc. 33: 1814-1824, 1974.
BARRY III, H. AND KRIMMER, E.C.: Discriminative stimulus effects of chlordiazepoxide related to general sedation. Communication at the Sixth International Congress of Pharmacology, Abstract no. 623, 1975.
COLPAERT, F.C.: Minireview. Narcotic cue and narcotic state. Life Sci. (in press), 1976.
COLPAERT, F.C., LAL, H., NIEMEGEERS, C.J.E. AND JANSSEN, P.A.J.: Investigations on drug produced and subjectively experienced discriminative stimuli. 1. The fentanyl

cue, a tool to investigate subjectively experienced narcotic drug actions. Life Sci. 16: 705-716, 1975a.
COLPAERT, F.C.: Apomorphine as a discriminative stimulus, and its antagonism by haloperidol. Eur. J. Pharmacol. 32: 383-386, 1975b.
COLPAERT, F.C., NIEMEGEERS, C.J.E. AND JANSSEN, P.A.J.: Differential response control by isopropamide: a peripherally induced discriminative cue. Eur. J. Pharmacol. 34: 381-384, 1975c.
COLPAERT, F.C., NIEMEGEERS, C.J.E. AND JANSSEN, P.A.J.: Theoretical and methodological considerations on drug discrimination learning. Psychopharmacologia 46: 169-177, 1976a.
COLPAERT, F.C., KUYPS, J.J.M.D., NIEMEGEERS, C.J.E. AND JANSSEN, P.A.J.: Discriminative stimulus properties of fentanyl and morphine: tolerance and dependence. Pharmacol. Biochem. Behav. (in press), 1976b.
COLPAERT, F.C., NIEMEGEERS, C.J.E. AND JANSSEN, P.A.J.: The narcotic discriminative stimulus complex: relation to analgesic activity. J. Pharm. Pharmacol. 28: 183-187, 1976c.
COLPAERT, F.C., DESMEDT, L.K.C. AND JANSSEN, P.A.J.: Discriminative stimulus properties of benzodiazepines, barbiturates and pharmacologically related drugs: relation to some intrinsic and anticonvulsant effects. Eur. J. Pharmacol. 37: 113-123, 1976d.
COLPAERT, F.C., NIEMEGEERS, C.J.E. AND JANSSEN, P.A.J.: Fentanyl and apomorphine: asymmetrical generalization of discriminative stimulus properties. Neuropharmacology (in press), 1976e.
COLPAERT, F.C., KUYPS, J.J.M.D., NIEMEGEERS, C.J.E. AND JANSSEN, P.A.J.: Discriminative stimulus properties of a low dl-amphetamine dose. Archs. Int. Pharmacodyn. Ther. (in press), 1976f.
COLPAERT, F.C., NIEMEGEERS, C.J.E., KUYPS, J.J.M.D AND JANSSEN, P.A.J.: Narcotic cue and narcotic state: differential involvement of brain 5-hydroxytryptamine. Neuropharmacology (in press), 1976g.
COLPAERT, F.C., VAN BEVER, W.F.M. AND LEYSEN, J.E.M.F.: Apomorphine: chemistry, pharmacology, biochemistry. Int. Rev. Neurobiol. 19: (in press), 1976h.
DEWS, P.B.: Are the techniques and results of studies of self-administration of drugs useful in other areas of psychobiology? Pharmacol. Rev. 27, 545-548, 1975.
DOTY, R.W. AND RUTLEDGE, L.T.: "Generalization" between cortically and peripherally applied stimuli eliciting conditioned reflexes. J. Neurophysiol. 22: 428-435, 1959.
GRILLY, D.M.: Effects of prior experience on differential learning under amphetamine. Psychopharmacologia 43: 271-277, 1975.

HEISE, G.A.: Discrete trial analysis of drug action. Fed. Proc. 34: 1898-1903, 1975.
HIRSCHHORN, I.D. AND ROSECRANS, J.A.: Morphine and 9-tetrahydrocannabinol: tolerance to the stimulus effects. Psychopharmacologia 36: 243-253, 1974.
JANSSEN, P.A.J., NIEMEGEERS, C.J.E. AND DONY, J.G.: The inhibitory effect of fentanyl (R 4263) and other morphine-like analgesics on the warm water-induced tail withdrawal reflex. Arzneim.-Forsch. 13: 502-507, 1963.
KUHN, D.M., GREENBERG, I. AND APPEL, J.B.: Stimulus properties of the narcotic antagonist pentazocine: similarity to morphine and antagonism by naloxone. J. Pharmacol. Exp. Ther. 196: 121-127, 1976.
MIGLER, B. AND MILLENSON, J.R.: Analysis of response rates during stimulus generalization. J. Exp. Anal. Behav. 12: 81-87, 1969.
OVERTON, D.A.: State-dependent or "dissociated" learning produced with pentobarbital. J. Comp. Physiol. Psychol. 57: 3-12, 1964.
OVERTON, D.A.: State-dependent learning produced by depressant and atropine-like drugs. Psychopharmacologia 10: 6-31, 1966.
OVERTON, D.A.: Dissociated learning in drug states (state dependent learning). In Psychopharmacology. A review of progress 1957-1967, ed. by D.H. Efron, J.O. Cole, J. Levine and J.R. Wittenborn, pp. 918-930, Public Health Service Publication No. 1836, U.S. Government Printing Office, Washington D.C., 1968.
OVERTON, D.A.: Discriminative control of behavior by drug states. In Stimulus properties of drugs, ed. by T. Thompson and R. Pickens, pp; 87-110, Appleton-Century-Crofts, New York, 1971.
OVERTON, D.A.: Experimental methods for the study of state-dependent learning. Fed. Proc. 33: 1800-1813, 1974.
RAY, B.A. AND SIDMAN, M.: Reinforcement schedules and stimulus control. In The theory of reinforcement schedules, ed. by W.N. Schoenfeld, pp. 187-214, Appleton-Century-Crofts, New York, 1970.
RILLING, M., CAPLAN, H.J., HOWARD, R.C. AND BROWN, C.H.: Inhibitory stimulus control following errorless discrimination learning. J. Exp. Anal. Behav. 24: 121-133, 1975.
ROFFMAN, M. AND LAL, H.: Role of brain amines in learning associated with "amphetamine-state". Psychopharmacologia 25: 195-204, 1972.
ROSECRANS, J.A., GOODLOE, M.H., BENNETT, G.J. AND HIRSCHHORN, I.D.: Morphine as a discriminative cue: effects of amine depletors and naloxone. Eur. J. Pharmacol. 21, 252-256, 1973.
SCHECHTER, M.D. AND ROSECRANS, J.A.: D-amphetamine as a discriminative cue: drugs with similar stimulus properties. Eur. J. Pharmacol. 21: 212-216, 1973.

WINTER, J.C.: A comparison of the stimulus properties of mescaline and 2, 3, 4-trimethoxyphenylethylamine. J.Pharmacol. Exp.Ther. 185: 101-107, 1973.
WINTER, J.C.: The effects of 3, 4-dimethoxyphenylethylamine in rats trained with mescaline as a discriminative stimulus. J.Pharmacol.Exp.Ther. 189: 741-747, 1974.
WINTER, J.C.: The stimulus properties of morphine and ethanol. Psychopharmacologia 44: 209-214, 1975.
WOODARD, W.T. AND BITTERMAN, M.E.: A discrete-trials/fixed-interval method of discrimination training. Behav. Res.Methods Instrum. 6: 389-392, 1974.

DISCRIMINABLE STIMULI PRODUCED BY ANALGESICS

Harbans Lal, Gerald Gianutsos and Stephen Miksic

Department of Pharmacology & Toxicology
and
Department of Psychology
University of Rhode Island
Kingston, R.I. 02881

I. INTRODUCTION

Narcotic analgesics are drugs primarily used to relieve pain. Although narcotic drugs were originally natural products, many new drugs are synthetic. All known narcotic analgesics also produce a number of effects other than analgesia which make them valuable for other clinical uses but also constitute potentials for abuse and narcotic dependence. In addition, there are several pharmacological properties which are characteristic of only a few narcotics and are absent in the rest of them. For example, morphine is known to initially cause vomiting and later show a strong anti-emetic property. All synthetic narcotics are purely anti-emetic and are devoid of the initial emetic action. Similarly, various narcotic analgesics differ in their respiratory depressant property. Whereas they all produce respiratory depression, with some a rapid tolerance develops which allows for further use to relieve pain without concomitant depression of respiration.

Narcotic analgesics act both centrally and peripherally. Whereas analgesia is due to an action in the central nervous system (CNS), inhibition of peristaltic reflexes is due to an action in the intestine. By virtue of their action on the intestine, the narcotics are potent antidiarrheal drugs (see Van Bever and Lal, 1976). However, this action of narcotic analgesics is not necessarily correlated with their potency as analgesics. Whereas some potent analgesics are poor antidiarrheals, other potent antidiarrheals are poor analgesics. Still others are equipotent as analgesics and antidiarrheals.

A property of narcotic analgesics which is intimately related to the abuse of narcotic analgesics is the euphoria typically produced by these drugs (Lal, 1976). Not enough is known to clearly define narcotic euphoria. It is considered to be a CNS mediated action which is subjectively perceived as a feeling of "unusual well being" that is incommensurate with the objective reality of the situation. Another property of this euphoria is that it produces a psychic drive that requires periodic or continuous administration of the drug to produce pleasure and avoid deprivation discomfort. According to Eddy et al.(1970) "this mental state is the most powerful of all the factors involved in chronic intoxication with psychotropic drugs, with certain types of drugs it may be the only factor involved, even in most intense craving and perpetuation of compulsive abuse".

Morphine (Hill et al. , 1971 ; Rosecrans et al. ,1973 ; Gianutsos and Lal, 1975 ; Shannon and Holtzman, 1976) and fentanyl (Colpaert et al.,1975a), two representative narcotic drugs, have been shown to produce a discriminable stimulus (DS) which controls behaviors. Animals can be trained to reliably emit one response when treated with the narcotic and an alternate response when treated with the vehicle. Therefore, it can be said that the pharmacological actions of narcotics produce an internal stimulus state which can be readily perceived and discriminated from the normal physiological state. What follows will describe in greater detail the properties of this discriminable stimulus state of narcotics and discuss its relationship with other pharmacological actions of these drugs.

II. PROCEDURES EMPLOYED

A number of procedures have been used to study discriminable drug-stimuli. Most of these procedures can be considered as variations of the three methods described below.

A. Free Operant Responding

The free operant was originally used to demonstrate the discrimination of alcohol from saline by Kubena and Barry (1969). In this procedure, rats are trained to press one lever after receiving the drug and a different lever after saline injection. In the last few years, a number of variations of this procedure have been introduced and are used in several laboratories. Below is a detailed description of a procedure which is routinely employed in our own laboratory.

1. Animals

Male hooded rats of the Long-Evans strain weighing 200-250 g at the start of the experiment are placed in single cages and adapted to consume their total daily ration of food (12-18 grams) within a few hours each afternoon (2-5 PM). Water is made continuously available. Nearly 2/3 of the rats adapt to this feeding schedule. The rats which do not adapt to this schedule within a week and begin to lose weight are discarded. The rats are housed in a room thermostatically maintained at 21°C. The room lights are turned off from 8 P.M. to 8 A.M.

2. Training

The behavioral apparatus consists of conventional Skinner boxes housed in sound attenuated chambers. The house lights remain on during the session. Each behavioral box contains two levers, one on either side of the food cup and equidistant from the center. All rats are first shaped to lever press for food reinforcement. As soon as they begin to lever press at a rate of 1/min they are shaped to learn a progressively increasing fixed ratio (FR) until they consistently respond on an FR10 schedule (10 lever presses for each 45 mg Noyes pellet). In the beginning, responding on one lever is reinforced while responding on the other lever is inconsequential. When the rat begins to respond on only one lever at an approximate rate of 20 responses a min the position of the correct lever is changed to the other side on the next day. Now the rat has to learn that the other lever is correct. After 4-5 such alternations without any injection, an injection schedule is introduced. In this phase of training, daily 15 min sessions are preceded by an injection of either the training drug (in this case, fentanyl or morphine) or the solvent for the drug, usually saline. After drug injection one lever is assigned to be the drug appropriate lever and only responses on this lever are reinforced. Alternatively, after saline injection only responses on the opposite lever (i.e., saline-appropriate) are reinforced. The other lever is made inconsequential. A possible effect of position preference is counterbalanced by randomly assigning the right lever to be the drug lever for half of the rats and the left lever to be the drug lever for the rest of the rats. For every individual rat the position (i.e. right or left) of the drug lever remains constant on subsequent sessions. In the beginning the rats receive either drug injection or a saline injection until responding is stabilized on the appropriate lever. Following this, the rat receives the alternate injection and must stabilize his responding on the opposite lever

until the new contingency is learned. The training is continued
until 10 alternations have been achieved. All rats reaching this
phase of training then enter into the final training phase where drug
injections are systematically alternated with saline injections
according to two weekly (5 days) alternating sequences. In one
week the sequence is saline-drug-drug-saline-saline. **In the following**
week, the sequence is drug-saline-saline-drug-drug. The two
sequences are alternated continuously as long as these rats are
used in these experiments. In this and in all subsequent phases
of the experiment, the session length is fixed at 10 min and the
data are recorded to include both the number of responses an
animal emits on each lever before the first reinforcement is
obtained and the total number of responses made during the whole
10 min session. The animals are considered adequately trained
when not more than 3 responses are made on the wrong lever
before 10 responses are made on the correct lever where the rat
is reinforced. In addition, the response rate should be more than
25/min. Even after the training the rats are constantly run without interruption on 5 days each week. This permits the rats to
improve their performance with time while they simultaneously
develop ever increasing resistance to extinction.

   3. Testing

      Once trained, the rats can be continuously and repeatedly
used for testing. Usually we designate Wednesday (or another 3rd
day if rats are not run daily) as test day. On this day the training
injection is replaced by an injection of the drug we are interested
in testing or the training drug at a different dose. According to
this schedule, in one week a training drug precedes the test day
while in the following week the test day is preceded by a saline day.
This way any after-effect of the pretest session is counter-balanced even though, up to the present time, we have not observed any
effect of the previous day's treatment on subsequent discrimination.
However, a long acting drug might interfere with responding on the
following day and in that case the rat is simply considered not
testable on that day. We have found that once adequately trained,
the discriminative responses are very resistant to extinction. This
conclusion is based upon our experiment in which, on certain days,
we switched the correct lever. A trained rat was injected with
the training drug but reinforced on what would ordinarily be the
saline appropriate lever. In this instance, the rats kept pressing
the drug appropriate lever in spite of not receiving any reinforcement. If the rat begins to press the other lever, he emits the rest
of the responses in that session on that lever. However, when
placed in the chamber again on the following day, these rats do not
show any effect of the new one-day learning they were exposed to

on the previous day. They always respond on the lever that had always been correct for an appropriate stimulus.

On the test day one of two procedures is followed. The rat is either left in the chamber until the first reinforcement is obtained or allowed to complete the whole session of 10 min as usual. In both cases, on the test day, responses on either lever are reinforced and the total number of responses emitted on each lever is recorded until the first reinforcement is obtained. In this way, the rat may make between 10-19 total responses before the first reinforcement is obtained (i.e. he may press one bar 10 times and the other bar 1-9 times until he receives his first reinforcement). The extent by which this number exceeds 10 directly reflects the disruption of discrimination. We found that the well trained rats rarely emit more than 14 total responses before the first reinforcement is obtained. As a matter of fact if a rat does make more than 14 responses on two sessions in a row we suspend that rat from testing and institute more training. As the trained rats do not exhibit trial and error behavior (i.e. pressing both levers) and they always emit 10 responses on the correct lever, the discrimination data can be easily considered all or none and processed directly for ED_{50} calculation.

Often, it is useful to determine if the test drug has other behavioral actions at the doses employed in the discrimination testing. If so, the effect on the rate of lever pressing can be determined in the same test session as described above. By permitting the rat to bar press for the complete 10 min the rate of emitted behavior can be easily obtained. The total number of bar presses will permit the investigator to calculate the operant rate under the influence of that drug. It offers an advantage to specify the relationship between a discriminable dose and the dose which affects behavior. Until now we have not found any such relationship. Rats will discriminate certain drugs at doses at which no effect on response rate is detected. In other cases the discriminable doses may either stimulate or depress operant responding.

B. Discrete Trial Responding

In this paradigm, the subject is allowed to make only one response on each trial. This response is either correct or incorrect. Either a Skinner box or a maze is used for discrete trial avoidance responding. Although drug discrimination has been achieved with the use of an appropriate maze paradigm, the most commonly used procedures for shock avoidance utilize a lever pressing response.

1. Lever Pressing Responses

The procedure used by Holtzman's group is best illustrated and represents typical features. A detailed description of this procedure will be given in Chapter 4 of this book. Briefly, three levers are used in conventional Skinner Boxes. Two response levers are on one wall of the chamber while a third "observing response lever" is on the opposite wall. A scrambled electric shock is delivered to the grid floor by a constant current shock generator. Rats are trained in a two-choice, discrete trial avoidance procedure to respond, on each trial, first on the observing lever and then on one of the two avoidance response levers to avoid or escape shock. During each training session, responses on one choice lever terminate a trial (the "appropriate" lever) and responses on the other lever (the "inappropriate" lever) do not have any consequence. During training sessions a trial is defined as being correct if the first discriminated response emitted by the animal following an observing response is on the appropriate lever However, during test sessions a response on either lever following an observing response terminates a trial (i.e., condition of non-differential reinforcement of choice responding). Training sessions and test sessions are identical in all other respects.

During each experimental session the beginning of a trial is signalled by the simultaneous onset of the houselight and white noise. The first observing response of each trial terminates the white noise; the houselight remains on until the appropriate choice response is made to terminate the trial. Beginning 5 sec after the onset of a trial a scrambled 1 mA electric shock is intermittently presented as 0.5 second pulses with 2.5 seconds between pulses for the duration of the trial. The first trial of every session serves as a "warm-up" and is not recorded. Once the rats are trained to a criterion of 18 out of 20 correct responses in 4-6 sessions, the test sessions are initiated when a test drug or dose is substituted for the training drug.

2. Maze Escape Response

Discrete trial escape responses in a T-maze have most often been used. This procedure for drug discrimination was first used by Stewart (1962). Briefly, rats are trained to escape from shock. On each trial the rat is placed in the starting place in one arm of the T-maze with the shock already turned on and is allowed to run freely in the maze until it reaches the correct goal box where the grid floor is without shock. Usually several trials are administered each day in a single session. The animal is required to turn into one side-arm under the drug and to the oppo-

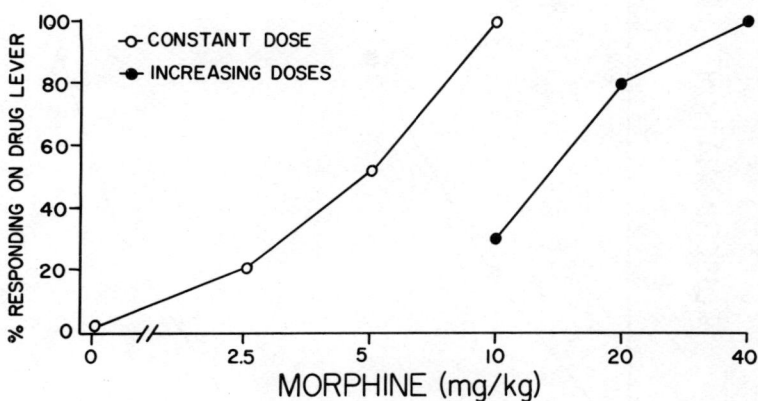

Figure 1

Dose-dependent elicitation of discriminable stimulus produced by morphine. Test doses of morphine were injected intraperitoneally into the rats previously trained to discriminate morphine (10 mg/kg) from saline. These rats (hollow circles) were considered as constant dose subjects (ED_{50}, 4.4 mg/kg). Solid circles represent data obtained after the rats were given systematically increasing doses of morphine sulfate to induce tolerance (increasing doses group; ED_{50} = 12.5 mg/kg). Percent of rats responding on the drug appropriate lever is given on Y-axis (adapted from Miksic and Lal, 1977).

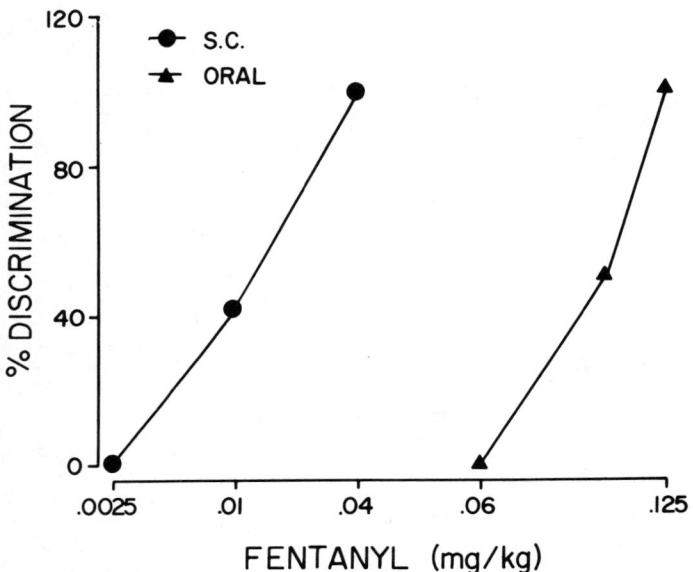

Figure 2

Dose-dependent elicitation of discriminable stimulus in rats produced by fentanyl. The rats were trained at a dose of 0.04 mg/kg given subcutaneously. The test dose was given either subcutaneously or orally. The percent of rats responding on narcotic appropriate lever is given on Y-axis. Data adapted from Colpaert et al., (1975a).

site side-arm of the maze under the saline. On the test day the rat selects one of the two responses based upon the perceived quality of stimulus induced by the injection.

This procedure is least sensitive in the sense that very high doses of a drug are necessary to impart discrimination training. It is usually used by investigators interested in state dependent learning.

III. DOSE RESPONSE CHARACTERISTICS

In order to establish that a measured effect of a drug actually represents a pharmacological action rather than some non-specific effect of drug administration, it is essential that dose dependency of this action is established. The DS produced by narcotics is a dose dependent action. Data summarized in Fig. 1 show the induction of DS produced by various doses of morphine in rats trained to discriminate morphine (10 mg/kg) from saline. Similarly, Shannon and Holtzman (1976) showed dose dependence with a number of narcotics tested. Data summarized in Fig. 2 show a dose response curve of the DS produced by fentanyl in rats trained to discriminate fentanyl (0.04 mg/kg) from saline. As is seen from these data, the DS produced by narcotics is a dose dependent action of these drugs. Also, the doses which are effective in producing DS are usually smaller than those producing other effects such as analgesia. In Table 1 are listed the effective doses of all drugs tested up until now. It is seen that in all cases the effective doses fall within the usual pharmacological range. It should be pointed out that the rats in which these doses are tested are usually tolerant to the analgesic action of narcotics. This question will be discussed later in this chapter. As ED_{50} values are not available for all compounds tested, ED_{100} values are given in Table 1. The available ED_{50} are given in Table 2. All of the narcotics produce DS in usual pharmacological doses.

IV. SPECIFICITY OF NARCOTIC STIMULUS

The DS produced by narcotics is specific to these drugs. It may be noted in Table 1 that all narcotics tested produced a positive DS similar to morphine or another narcotic used as a training drug. They included naturally occurring as well as synthetic analgesics and belonged to several chemical classes. Moreover, enuntiomorphs of same narcotics were inactive. For example, whereas levorphanol is active in producing a narcotic DS, a dose 30 fold higher of its sterio-isomer, dextrophan is inactive. The l-isomer is similarly more active as an analgesic.

Table 1. ED_{100}[1] values for different narcotics in narcotic discrimination tests

Training			Testing		
Drug	mg/kg	Route	Drug	Route	ED_{100}
Morphine	10	IP	Morphine	IP	10
				Oral	50
			Methadone	IP	4
			Fentanyl	IP	0.32
			Propoxyphene	IP	25
	3	S.C.	Morphine	SC	3
			Methadone	"	3
			Isomethadone	"	3
			Meperidine	"	30
			Codeine	"	30
			Propoxyphene	"	30
			Alphaprodine	"	1
			Heroin	"	1
			Levorphanol	"	1
			Oxymorphanol	"	1
			Oxymorphone	"	0.3
			Phenazocine	"	0.1
			Fentanyl	"	0.03
			Etonitazine	"	0.003
			Butorphanol	"	0.3
			Nalmexone	"	10
Fentanyl	0.04	S.C.	Cyclazocine	"	0.31
			Dextromoramide	"	0.63
			Fentanyl	"	0.04
			Methadone	"	2.5
			Pentazocine	"	20
			Meperidine	"	10
			Morphine	"	10
			Phenoperidine	"	0.31
			Piritramide	"	5
			Sulfentanil	"	0.0025
Fentanyl	1.25	Oral	Bezitramide	Oral	1.25
			Codeine	"	40
			Dextromoramide	"	2.5
			Diphenoxylate	"	20
			Fentanyl	"	1.25
			Methadone	"	20
			Morphine	"	40
			Meperidine	"	40

[1] Values for fentanyl trained rats were provided by F. Colpaert, and those for morphine 3 mg/kg were provided by S. Holtzman.

Another test for specificity is the remarkable antagonism of the DS by specific narcotic antagonists. The DS produced by narcotics is antagonized by small doses of naloxone (Gianutsos and Lal, 1976) and naltrexone (Shannon and Holtzman, 1977). These data will be discussed in another chapter in detail.

Table 2. ED_{50} values for orally administered narcotic analgesics in drug discrimination tests and tail withdrawal tests[1]

	ED_{50} (mg/kg, P.O.)		
Drug	DS	Mild Analgesic	Pronounced Analgesic
Benzitramide	0.57	0.38	0.88
Fentanyl	0.63	0.42	1.14
Dextromoramide	1.78	1.98	3.29
Diphenoxine	3.40	2.57	17
Diphenoxylate	7.10	6.90	27
Methadone	8.50	13.50	17
Morphine	20	14	33
Codeine	23	19	56
Propoxyphene	36	65	65

[1] Extrapolated from data of Niemegeers et al., (1976).

Further evidence for the specificity of action is that there is a perfect correlation between the ED_{50} values for analgesia and those for DS in all tested compounds varying greatly in their potency. Data summarized in Table 2 give ED_{50} values for both analgesia and DS. An almost perfect correlation in the rank order is evident. Also in Table 3 are given the relative potency of each narcotic in producing DS and similar potency in producing analgesia in human patients. Again, a remarkable similarity in the rank order is evident.

Based upon the structure-activity relationship, antagonism by specific narcotic antagonists and the high correlation between analgesic potency and DS, it can be stated with certainty that the DS produced by narcotic analgesics is a highly specific action of this class of drugs, as much as the analgesic action of these drugs is.

Table 3. Relative potency of narcotic analgesics in producing discriminable stimuli and analgesia[1]

Drug	Discriminative Stimulus (rat)	Analgesia (man)
Sulfentanil	4000	-
Etonitazine	1000	-
Fentanyl	100	80
Oxymorphone	10	10
Phenazocine	10	3
Levorphanol	3	3
Heroin	3	3
Alphaprodine	3	0.25
Methadone	2	1
Morphine	1	1
Isomethadone	1	0.3
Meperidine	0.1	0.1
Codeine	0.1	0.1
Propoxyphene	0.02	-

[1] Data provided by Holtzman and Niemegeers were extrapolated and approximated when necessary.

V. SITE OF ACTION

Since narcotic drugs produce both central and peripheral actions, both of which consist of marked physiological changes, it is interesting to know whether the DS is based upon a central or peripheral action. There are several lines of evidence to indicate that the DS is produced through a central action.

The major peripheral action of narcotic analgesics is the inhibition of the intestinal reflex. In whole animals this is usually tested by inhibition of castor oil-induced diarrhea. Data summarized in Table 4 show that all narcotics are more potent antidiarrheals than analgesics. There are also structurally related antidiarrheals which are much more potent antidiarrheals than analgesics. Whereas the highest separation between the analgesic and antidiarrheal potency of narcotics is only 20 fold, synthetic antidiarrheals are nearly 100 fold more potent in inhibiting diarrhea than in reducing pain. This separation between these two effects is almost complete in newer antidiarrheals such as loperamide and fluperamide. These drugs in doses more than a thousand times higher than the effective antidiarrheal dose do not produce analgesia. Therefore by testing the potency of the narcotic DS, it is possible to determine if the DS is more closely related to analgesia or to the action of the drug on intestinal smooth muscle.

Table 4. A comparison of analgesic and anti-diarrheal potency of representative analgesics and antidiarrheals

Drug	Minimum ED_{50}		
	Analgesic	Antidiarrheal	Ratio
Analgesics			
Benzitramide	0.88	0.26	3.4
Fentanyl	1.14	0.19	6.0
Dextromoramide	3.29	1.80	1.8
Phenazocine	8.9	6.65	1.3
Anilaridine	11.6	4.42	2.6
Methadone	16.9	2.19	7.7
Phenoperidine	26.9	8.70	3.1
Piritramide	32.9	1.97	16.7
Morphine	33.6	1.52	22.1
Codeine	56.6	2.85	19.8
Demerol	63.5	16.30	3.9
Antidiarrheals			
Difenoxin	4.1	0.04	102
Butoxylate	13.6	0.13	105
Diphenoxylate	12.8	0.15	85
Fluperamide	160	0.15	1067
Loperamide	160	0.15	1067

[1] Extrapolated from Niemegeers et al., (1976).

Data summarized in Table 2 give the ED_{50} values for antidiarrheals in producing narcotic-like DS. Loperamide tested in oral doses up to 160 mg/kg and systemic doses up to 20 mg/kg did not produce any detectable narcotic DS (Gianutsos and Lal, 1975; Colpaert et al., 1975a). Two other antidiarrheals which produce narcotic DS do so in doses 50 fold higher than those producing inhibition of intestinal peristalsis. It is seen that drugs which have only peripheral narcotic-like activity, and do not act in the CNS, remarkably do not produce a morphine-like DS. Diphenoxylate and diphenoxine, which do produce a DS, do so only at doses which are analgesic and are many-fold higher than their effective antidiarrheal doses. Similarly, some narcotics produce a DS only at doses which are higher than their antidiarrheal ED_{50}. Whereas there is a perfect correlation between analgesic ED_{50} and DS ED_{50} of narcotics, there is no such correlation between antidiarrheal ED_{50} and DS ED_{50} in all of the drugs tested to date. Therefore, it can be concluded that an action in the intestine, no matter how potent it may be, does not constitute a DS which controls behavior.

Another line of evidence is also important to examine. A particular drug has different potency depending upon the route of administration. Most narcotics are less active as analgesics when administered orally. Therefore, we can examine the DS associated with narcotics when given both orally and systemically. Data summarized in Table 1 show that both in the case of morphine and fentanyl, the oral doses which produce a DS are several times higher than their systemic doses and are proportional to the oral/systemic difference in their analgesic potency. The same is not true when their antidiarrheal potency is examined. Whereas the antidiarrheal potency is increased when drugs are given orally, their DS producing activity is considerably decreased by this route of administration.

The dose response relationship between oral and systemic doses of fentanyl producing narcotic DS can be examined from data illustrated in Fig. 2.

VI. ROLE OF ANALGESIA AND TOLERANCE

Data summarized in Table 2 show ED_{50} values obtained by measuring DS and analgesia. The analgesia was measured by a tail withdrawal procedure of Janssen et al., (1963). In this procedure, the rat is held in a rat holder with his tail freely hanging out of the holder. The tip of the tail is dipped up to 5 cm in water kept at 55°C. The time of tail withdrawal out of water is noted. The analgesia is usually defined at two levels. Mild but

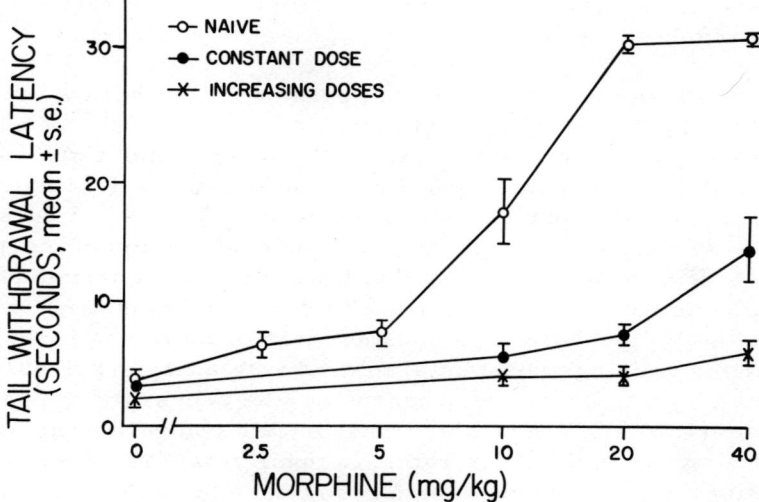

Figure 3

Morphine-induced analgesia in rats following onset of tolerance at different levels. One group of rats was given morphine at a constant dose of 10 mg/kg, 2-3 times per week for 8-12 weeks. These rats were then given systematically increasing doses of morphine until a daily dose of 100 mg/kg was reached in 10 days. Data adapted from Miksic and Lal (1977).

definite analgesia was defined as induction of tail withdrawal latency to 6 sec or above. This magnitude of latency is present only in 2.4% of animals treated with saline (Janssen et al., 1963). The tail withdrawal latency after saline is only 3-4 seconds. Marked analgesia was defined as latency of greater than 10 sec which is never found in an untreated rat. It is seen that the ED_{50} for the DS is similar to doses producing mild analgesia and is lower than ED_{50} values for marked analgesia. It may be pointed out that the analgesia data were obtained in rats which had not previously received morphine, whereas the DS measurements were made in rats treated with a constant dose of narcotic 2-3 times a week for several weeks. In order to obtain a relationship between analgesia and the DS the data obtained from the same rats may also be reviewed.

The data summarized in Figure 3 show tail-withdrawal latency as affected by different doses of morphine, at different intensities of tolerance. In naive rats, a dose of 5 mg/kg of morphine caused pronounced analgesia (7.88 ± 0.9 secs) so that the tail-withdrawal latency was nearly doubled (baseline latency = 3.58 ± 0.3 secs, $t(22) = 4.70$ $P<.01$). As expected, the analgesic action of morphine was dose dependent. It is seen that tolerance rapidly developed to the analgesic potency of morphine. In the experimental rats, intermittently injected with a constant dose of morphine for discrimination training, substantial tolerance to analgesia is observed. A dose as high as 20 mg/kg of morphine was necessary to produce analgesia (7.70 ± 0.7 sec) which was roughly comparable to a dose of 5 mg/kg in the naive rats. In these rats, treatment with increasing doses of morphine induced further tolerance so that even a dose of 40 mg/kg was ineffective in producing significant analgesia.

In spite of complete tolerance to analgesia at a test dose of 10 mg/kg, the discrimination trained rats showed a completely accurate perception of the DS. At this dose all rats in all test trials recognized the morphine stimulus reliably, even though they failed to produce analgesia. As shown in Figure 3, the rats who were made systematically tolerant to the analgesic action of morphine showed a characteristic dose dependence of the discrimination of morphine. When the rats were rendered highly tolerant by increasing doses of morphine, the sensitivity to morphine's analgesic action was completely lost. However, these rats still showed a dose dependent perception of the morphine-induced discriminable stimulus at which, using other tests, the animal would appear completely tolerant.

As in the case of other actions of morphine, injection of incremental doses produced tolerance to the DS produced by morphine. In Figure 1 it can be seen that the dose-response curve of morphine DS is shifted to the right. Whereas all rats recognized the 10 mg/kg dose as morphine prior to development of high tolerance, only 4 of 12 demonstrated this recognition after treatment with increasing doses of morphine. This difference was highly significant ($X^2 = 69$, $P<0.001$).

The data summarized in Table 5 show that there was no difference in tail withdrawal latency between the rats who recognized the DS and those who did not. In both groups the tail withdrawal latency was shorter than the 6 seconds considered necessary to reflect analgesia. This suggests that the recognition of the morphine DS is not contingent upon perception of the analgesic action of morphine.

Table 5. Tail withdrawal latency (seconds) of morphine tolerant rats injected with different doses of morphine (Miksic and Lal, 1977).

Morphine (mg/kg)	Tail withdrawal latency, Mean ± S.E.	
	Morphine Responding Rats	Saline Responding Rats
10	4.5 ± 0.6	4.1 ± 0.6
20	3.8 ± 0.8	4.6 ± 11
40	4.0 ± 1.0	-

It is clear from these data that tolerance develops to the DS producing action of morphine. Shannon and Holtzman (1976) have found similar tolerance when they measured the numbers of responses made on the drug appropriate lever by the DS trained rats. It seems that perception of morphine DS is not dependent upon the analgesic action of morphine, as this DS can be perceived even by rats fully tolerant to analgesia. Also, it can be concluded from these data that the subjects show a markedly higher sensitivity to the perception of the DS than to the analgesic action of narcotics. Moreover, the perception of DS does not depend on the perception of analgesia. The rats seem to learn to perceive the DS produced by narcotics even when analgesia is not present. Therefore, the neuronal substrates of the DS produced by narcotics, and those for narcotic analgesia, must be different, at least with respect to their perception sensitivity. It may also be concluded that the subjects are not discriminating narcotics because of their

analgesic property. This view is supported by the fact that the
perception of morphine DS was not correlated with tail withdrawal latency, a very reliable measure of analgesia. A previous
report (Colpaert et al, 1976) of a high correlation between analgesia
and DS was based upon analgesia measurements performed in
naive rats where analgesic doses of narcotics are expected to be
far lower than those expected from the tolerant rats, as is shown
in the experiment reported here.

VII. MECHANISM OF ACTION

The precise mechanism for the narcotic DS has not been
clearly established. Whereas the narcotic DS is readily generalized to a large number of narcotic drugs (see Section IV.), there is
no generalization to any other non-narcotic compound thus far
tested, as seen in Table 6, whose mechanisms are better understood. For instance, amphetamine (Roffman and Lal, 1972) and
apomorphine (Colpaert et al.,1975b) both are capable of producing
a DS and apparently do so by a mechanism involving increased
activity of dopaminergic systems (Ho and Huang, 1975; Colpaert
et al.,1975b). However, neither compound is perceived as a drug
in rats trained to make a morphine-saline discrimination
(Gianutsos and Lal, 1976) or a fentanyl-saline discrimination
(Colpaert et al., 1975a). Similarly, neither pharmacological agents
known to act via acetylcholine, norepinephrine, or serotonin nor
non-specific CNS depressants are capable of eliciting a narcotic
response in trained rats. These results are illustrated in Table
6. It is evident that morphine either produces a DS through some
other neurotransmitter or more likely, that the stimulus is not
produced through a simple action involving only one transmitter
substance.

To further test the mechanism involved, the ability of various
compounds to antagonize the narcotic DS has been investigated.
If, for example, a drug with a known mechanism of action is
capable of disrupting the DS produced by morphine in a trained rat
it may provide a clue for the pharmacological actions involved in
producing the DS. As previously noted in Section IV, narcotic
antagonists are very active in counteracting the cue produced by
narcotics as well as the more classical actions of narcotics.
Recent experiments would suggest, however, that this capacity is
unique for narcotic antagonists since a number of non-narcotic
compounds were tested (amphetamine, p-chloramphetamine,
apomorphine, haloperidol, pilocarpine, dexetimide, cyproheptadine,
propranolol) and found to be inactive in antagonizing the morphine
DS, (Gianutsos and Lal, 1976). These compounds were tested at
various doses which included those high enough to completely

suppress bar-pressing behavior. The wide spectrum of action of these tested compounds further argues against a simple mechansim for the narcotic DS.

Table 6. Drugs which stimulate responding on saline lever in the rats trained to discriminate narcotics from saline[1]

Drug	Highest Dose Tested
Acetylsalicylic Acid	160
Amphetamine	3.2
Apomorphine	1.25
Atropine	5
Azaperone	2.5
Caffeine	20
Chlorpromazine	2.5
Clonidine	2.5
Cocaine	10
Cyclazocine (some tests)	3
Cyproheptadine	8
Desipramine	20
Dextimide	0.64
Dextrorphan	30
Haloperidol	0.64
Imipramine	40
Indomethacin	10
Isopropamide	0.32
Ketamine	30
Ketocyclazocine	3
Levallorphan	30
Librium	5
L-Methyl-p-tyrosine	200
Loperamide	20
LSD	0.08
Mescaline	100
Nalbuphine	100
Nalorphine	40
Naloxone	16
Naltrexone	3
Nicotine	0.16
Oxilorphan	30
P-chloramphetamine	12
Pentobarbital	20
Phenacetin	160
Phenylbutazone	160
Physostigmine	1

Pilocarpine	4
Scopolamine	1
Spipeperone	0.08
Suprofan	160
Thebaine	10
Tolmetin	160

[1] Data taken from several investigators (Colpaert et al., 1975c; Gianutsos and Lal, 1976; Shannon and Holtzman, 1976; unpublished data from Lal).

It should be pointed out that the morphine DS differs from other behavioral effects associated with narcotics. The self-administration of morphine is blocked by haloperidol (Hansen and Cimini-Venoma, 1973; Gianutsos and Lal, 1975), spiramide (Lal and Hynes, 1977), and by methyl tyrosine (Pozuelo and Kerr, 1972) a compound which inhibits the synthesis of catecholamines (Spector et al., 1965). These drugs and several additional compounds representing other pharmacological classes also suppress the withdrawal symptoms observed during narcotic abstinence (Lal and Numan, 1976; Lal and Hynes, 1977). None of these drugs either substitute for or block narcotic DS. Thus, there seems to be a separation between the subjective effects of narcotics on one hand and the reinforcing properties and abstinence blockade on the other hand.

It appears fairly certain, therefore, that the narcotic cue, although highly specific, is not the result of a simple mechanism, and is not due to dopaminergic, cholinergic or serotonergic systems acting independently. It is possible that morphine may interact with an endogenous factor which produces alterations at several levels of the CNS, all of which may interact and contribute to the subjective perception of a drug as a narcotic.

Although narcotic DS cannot be produced by any other drug, it can be elicited by a conditional stimulus (Miksic et al., 1976) which has previously been proposed to release endorphin (Lal et al., 1976).

VIII. RESEARCH AND CLINICAL APPLICATIONS

The drug discrimination paradigm has several potentially useful applications in basic and therapeutic research. They have been discussed elsewhere (Lal, this book). Thus far only other narcotic agonists have been shown to substitute for a narcotic DS in a trained rat and the stimulus has been antagonized only by known narcotic antagonists. For this reason, it provides a screening procedure for detecting drugs with narcotic agonist or antagonist properties. A newly synthesized compound could be injected into rats trained to discriminate morphine from vehicle. If the rats make drug-appropriate responses, it could be predicted that the compound would be an effective narcotic-like analgesic in man. Testing of the potency of the compound relative to morphine could provide a basis for its effective clinical dose. Likewise, the duration of action could be similarly tested. In an analagous manner, drugs could be screened for narcotic antagonist properties if they cause a morphine treated rat to respond on the vehicle-appropriate bar.

In addition, this procedure may be useful in evaluating the potential for abuse of a new compound. A novel analgesic which does not cause a trained rat to bar press on the narcotic-appropriate lever would probably not produce narcotic-like subjective effects and would therefore not be subject to abuse of narcotic type. Similarly, an analysis of the mechanisms and brain areas involved in producing DS may shed some light on the physiology of the subjective effects of narcotics and possibly the "high" produced by the drugs.

IX. REFERENCES

Colpaert, F.C., Lal, H., Niemegeers, C.J.E. and Janssen, P.A.J.: Investigations on drug produced and subjectively experienced discriminative stimuli. I. The fentanyl cue, a tool to investigate subjectively experienced narcotic drug actions. Life Sci. 16: 705-716, 1975a.

Colpaert, F.C., Niemegeers, C.J.E., Kuyps, J.J.M.D. and Janssen, P.A.J.: Apomorphine as a discriminative stimulus and its antagonism by haloperidol. Eur. J. Pharmacol. 32: 383-386, 1975b.

Colpaert, F.C., Niemegeers, C.J.E. and Janssen, P.A.J.: The narcotic cue: evidence for the specificity of the stimulus properties of narcotic drugs. Arch. Int. Pharmacodyn. Ther. 218: 268-276, 1975c.

Colpaert, F.C., Niemegeers, C.J.E. and Janssen, P.A.J.: The narcotic discriminative stimulus complex: relation to analgesic activity. J. Pharm. Pharmacol. 28: 183-187, 1976.

Eddy, N.B., Hallach, H., Isabell, H. and Seevers, M.H.: Drug dependence: its significance and characteristics. In Drug Abuse, Data and Debate, ed. by P. H. Blaeky, Thomas,

Springfield, 1970.

Gianutsos, G. and Lal, H.: Effect of loperamide, haloperidol and methadone in rats trained to discriminate morphine from saline. Psychopharmacol. 41: 267-270, 1975.

Gianutsos, G. and Lal, H.: Selective interaction of drugs with a discriminable stimulus associated with narcotic action. Life Sci. 19: 91-98, 1976.

Hanson, H.M. and Cimini-Venoma, C.A.: Effect of haloperidol on self-administration of morphine in rats. Fed. Proc. 3: 503, 1972.

Hill, H.E., Jones, B.E. and Bell, E.C.: State dependent control of discrimination by morphine and pentobarbital. Psychopharmacol. 22: 305-313, 1971.

Ho, B.T. and Huang, J.T.: Role of dopamine in d-amphetamine induced discrimination responding. Pharmacol. Biochem. Behav. 3: 1085-1092, 1975.

Janssen, P.A.J., Niemegeers, C.J.E. and Dony, J.G.H.: The inhibitory effect of fentanyl and other morphine-like analgesics on the warm water induced tail withdrawal reflex in rats. Arzneimittel-Forschung 13: 502-507, 1963.

Kubena, R.K. and Barry, H.: Two procedures for training differential responses in alcohol and non-drug conditions. J. Pharmaceut. Sci. 58: 99-101, 1969.

Lal, H., Miksic, S. and Smith, N.: Naloxone antagonism of conditioned hyperthermia: An evidence for release of endogenous opioid. Life Sci. 18: 971-976, 1976.

Lal, H.: Facts and falacies of addiction liability and abuse potentials. In Synthetic Antidiarrheal Drugs, ed. by W. Van Bever and H. Lal, pp. 235-251, Marcel Dekker Inc., New York, 1976.

Lal, H. and Hynes, M.D.: Effectiveness of butyrophenones and related drugs in narcotic withdrawal. Proc. 10th CINP Congress 1977, in press.

Lal, H. and Numan, R.: Blockade of morphine-withdrawal body shakes by haloperidol. Life Sci. 18: 163-168, 1976.

Miksic, S. and Lal, H.: Conditioning of discriminable stimuli produced by morphine. Psychopharmacol. Comm., 1976, in press.

Miksic, S. and Lal, H.: Tolerance to morphine produced discriminative stimuli and analgesia. Psychopharmacol., 1977, in press.

Niemegeers, C., Lenaerts, F. and Awouters, F.: In vivo pharmacology of antidiarrheal drugs. In Synthetic Antidiarrheal Drugs, Ed. by W. Van Bever and H. Lal, pp. 65-114, Marcel Dekker, Inc., 1976.

Pozuelo, J. and Kerr, F.W.L.: Suppression of craving and other signs of dependence in morphine-addicted monkeys by administration of alpha-methyl-para-tyrosine. Mayo Clinic Proc. 47: 621-625, 1972.

Roffman, M. and Lal, H.: Role of brain amines in learning associated with amphetamine state. Psychopharmacol. 25: 195-204, 1972.

Rosecrans, J.A., Goodloe, M.H., Bennet, G.J. and Hirschorn, I.D.: Morphine as a discriminative cue: Effects of amine depletors and naloxone. Eur. J. of Pharmacol. 21: 252-256, 1973.

Shannon, H.E. and Holtzman, S.G.: Evaluation of the discriminative effects of morphine in the rat. J. Pharmacol. and Exp. Therap. 198: 54-65, 1976.

Shannon, H.E. and Holtzman, S.G.: Blockade of the discriminative effects of morphine in the rat by naltrexone and naloxone. Psychopharmacol., 1977, in press.

Spector, S., Sjoedesma, A. and Udenfriend, A.: Blockade of norepinephrine synthesis by a-methyl-p-tyrosine, an inhibitor of tyrosine hydroxylase. J. Pharmacol. Exp. Therap. 147: 86-95, 1965.

Stewart, J.: Differential responses based on physiological consequences of pharmacological agents. Psychopharmacol. 3: 132-138, 1962.

Van Bever, W. and Lal, H. eds.: Synthetic Antidiarrheal Drugs, Marcel Dekker, Inc., 1976.

DISCRIMINATIVE PROPERTIES OF NARCOTIC ANTAGONISTS

Stephen G. Holtzman, Harlan E. Shannon and Gerald J. Schaefer

Department of Pharmacology
Emory University
Atlanta, Georgia 30322

I. INTRODUCTION

There have been many recent reports characterizing the discriminative properties of morphine and related narcotic analgesics in a variety of experimental paradigms, predominantly in the rat (see preceding chapter). It is becoming increasingly evident that a strong association exists between the discriminative properties of these drugs in animals and the qualitative nature of the subjective effects produced by these same drugs in man (Shannon and Holtzman, 1976a, b). Since the abuse potential of narcotic analgesics is largely a function of the nature of their subjective effects (see Fraser, 1968; Jasinski, 1973a), animal models for evaluating this component of drug action are of obvious importance on clinical as well as on theoretical grounds.

The observations that nalorphine is an effective analgesic in man (Lasagna and Beecher, 1954) and yet engenders little physical dependence or priminent drug-seeking behavior (Isbell, 1956; Martin and Gorodetzky, 1965) spurred the development of numerous analgesics with mixed agonist and narcotic antagonist properties (see reviews by Archer and Harris, 1965; Martin, 1967; Villarreal, 1970, 1973; Lewis et al., 1971). An extensive series of studies at the Addiction Research Center in Lexington, Kentucky, subsequently resulted in the identification and characterization of two distinct syndromes of subjective effects that are produced by narcotic-antagonist analgesics (Jasinski, 1973a; Haertzen, 1974).

At one extreme are drugs such as profadol and propiram which produce euphoric subjective effects that are qualitatively indistinguishable from those produced by morphine (Jasinski et al., 1971). The other end of the spectrum is represented by the nalorphine-cyclazocine-type compounds that produce dysphoric subjective disturbances ranging from tiredness and drunkeness to disorientation and psychotomimetic phenomena (Martin et al., 1965; Haertzen, 1970). Midway on this continuum are numerous compounds, such as pentazocine, butorphanol and nalbuphine, which exhibit a mixture of agonist properties of both the morphine and cyclazocine types (Jasinski et al., 1970; Jasinski and Mansky, 1972; Jasinski et al., 1975) and, consequently, cannot be assigned exclusively to either of those two classes of narcotic antagonists. As in the case of the narcotic analgesics, the abuse potential of the narcotic antagonists is also closely related to the type of subjective effects that they occasion (Jasinsky, 1973a,b). Thus, the greatest potential for abuse resides in the morphine-like antagonists whereas the abuse potential of the cyclazocine-like compounds is nil; drugs such as pentazocine again hold a position between the extremes.

Any animal model from which experimental findings are to be extrapolated to man with a measure of confidence must be able to provide data from which accurate predictions can be made over the broadest range of drug conditions that can be imposed. Accordingly, the narcotic antagonists would seem to present a special challenge in the development and validation of drug discrimination models for the prediction of the subjective effects of analgesics in man by virtue of the fact that antagonists are known to produce a broad spectrum of subjective effects, and yet still have many other actions in common among themselves as well as with morphine and related narcotic analgesics. These include, in addition to analgesia, respiratory depression, depression of polysynaptic spinal reflexes, depression of the twitch response of the electrically stimulated guinea pig ileum, pupillary constriction, effects on endocrine systems, and the capacity to induce tolerance and physical dependence (see Martin, 1967).

Two approaches have been followed in characterizing the discriminative properties of narcotic antagonists. The first, and predominant one, has been to test narcotic antagonists for stimulus generalization characteristics in animals trained to discriminate between a narcotic analgesic and its vehicle. The other approach has been to conduct tests of stimulus generalization in animals trained to discriminate between a narcotic antagonist and drug vehicle. As in the case of studies of the discriminative properties of narcotic analgesics, the rat has served as the test subject for most studies involving narcotic antagonists. More recently, Schaefer and Holtzman (1976) initiated a series of experiments to extend observations to a second species, the squirrel monkey. The behavioral base lines for studying the discriminative properties of narcotic antagonists have ranged from free operant responding maintained by food reinforcement to discrete trial avoidance paradigms.

II. DISCRIMINATION PROCEDURES

Rat.

Several investigators (e.g., Gianutsos and Lal, 1975, 1976; Colpaert et al., 1976) have used a two-choice 10-response fixed ratio (FR10) schedule of food reinforcement. Under this procedure the animals are injected with the training drug or drug vehicle then placed into a test chamber with two response manipulanda. One lever is appropriate for the drug condition and the other for the vehicle condition. Every tenth response on the appropriate lever results in the delivery of a food pellet. Acquisition of the discrimination is considered to have occurred when the animals reliably emit the first ten responses of a session on the appropriate lever. The degree to which the animals generalize their training conditions to test drugs is assessed either in terms of the percent of the first ten responses of the test that are emitted on the drug appropriate lever (Gianutsos and Lal, 1975, 1976) or in terms of the percent of animals that complete the first FR10 of the session on the drug-appropriate lever (Colpaert et al., 1976). Rats have been trained to discriminate between saline and 10 mg/kg of morphine injected i.p. 45 min before the start of an experimental session (Gianutsos and Lal, 1975, 1976), and between drug vehicle and 0.04 mg/kg of fentanyl administered subcutaneously 30 min before a session (Colpaert et al., 1976).

Kuhn et al., (1976) trained rats to discriminate between saline and 10 mg/kg of pentazocine injected intraperitoneally (30 min pretreatment) in a two-choice procedure in which the completion of a 10-response fixed ratio at the end of a variable interval averaging one min (tandem VI1FR10) resulted in the delivery of water reinforcement. A lever in one wall of the chamber was appropriate for the pentazocine condition and a lever in the opposite wall was appropriate for the saline condition. The accuracy of the discrimination was determined during variable-length extinction periods at the start of each session on the basis of the percentage of the total number of responses emitted in that period that were made on the appropriate lever. The stimulus properties of test drugs were evaluated in a similar manner during a 5-min extinction period at the start of the experimental session.

Shannon and Holtzman (1976a, b) have developed a modified two-choice discrete trial avoidance paradigm in which the animal is required to complete a two-response chain in order to terminate the trial and avoid or escape from electric shocks delivered to the grid floor of the experimental chamber. The start of a trial is signalled by illumination of the house light at which time the animal must first press a single response lever mounted in one wall of the chamber, then move to the opposite wall of the chamber and press one of the two choice response levers mounted therein. Morphine (3.0 mg/kg) or saline were administered subcutaneously 30 min prior to a training session. Half of the animals were trained to press the right choice lever throughout each morphine session and the left choice lever throughout the saline sessions; the other half of the animals were trained under the opposite conditions. Each experimental session consisted of 21 trials and the animals were trained until they could reliably complete 90% of the last 20 trials on the appropriate choice lever (the first trial of the session was considered to be a "warm-up" trial and was excluded from the data collection). When acquisition of the discrimination was completed, drug test sessions were interposed between training sessions. During training sessions only a response on the appropriate choice lever terminated a trial; a trial could be terminated by a response on either choice lever during drug tests. A test drug was considered to produce discriminative effects which were equivalent to those produced by the training dose of morphine if an average of at least 90% of the 20 trials of the drug test session were completed on the morphine-appropriate choice lever.

Squirrel Monkey.

The procedure for training and testing the squirrel monkeys (Schaefer and Holtzman, 1976) is basically similar to that employed by Shannon and Holtzman (1976a, b) with the rat. The monkeys were restrained in a primate cockpit and trained in a discrete trial avoidance procedure to press one of two choice levers in order to prevent or terminate the delivery of an electric shock to the tail. (Only a single lever response was required in contrast to the two-response chain used for the rats.) One group of monkeys was trained to discriminate between saline and 3.0 mg/kg of morphine; a second group was trained on a vehicle vs. 0.1 mg/kg of cyclazocine discrimination. Drugs were injected intramuscularly 15 min before the start of a 25-trial session. When the monkeys could reliably complete 88% of the trials (i.e., 22 out of 25) on the appropriate lever, drug test sessions were interposed between training sessions. During training sessions a trial could be terminated only by a response on the "correct" (i.e., appropriate) lever; a response on the incorrect lever had no programmed consequences. During drug test sessions both choice levers were activated so that the first response on either lever terminated the trial. A test drug was considered to produce discriminative effects which were equivalent to those produced by the training drug if an average of at least 88% of the trials of a test session were completed on the drug-appropriate choice lever.

III. DISCRIMINATIVE PROPERTIES IN THE RAT

Dose-Response Relationships

Holtzman and Shannon (1976a, b) tested ten narcotic antagonists in rats trained on the saline vs. morphine discrimination. Of those, four produced discriminative effects that were comparable to morphine's. The dose-response curves of three of these drugs-butorphanol, profadol and pentazocine-are compared with the morphine dose-response curve in Fig. 1. It can be seen that an average of at least 90% of the trials were completed on the morphine-appropriate choice lever following the administration of the training dose of morphine (3.0 mg/kg), 0.3 mg/kg of butorphanol, 3.0 mg/kg of profadol and 10 mg/kg of pentazocine. Nalmexone, which is not illustrated in Fig. 1, was tested over a dose range of 0.1 - 10 mg/kg; trails completed on the morphine-appropriate choice lever average 92 and 98% after the administration of 3.0 and 10 mg/kg, respectively. The relative potencies for producing morphine-like discriminative effects can be estimated by considering the lowest dose of each drug which produced at least 90% responding on the morphine-appropriate choice lever. If 3.0 mg/kg of morphine is assigned a potency of 1, the potencies of the narcotic antagonists relative to morphine would range from 10 for butorphanol to 0.33 for pentazocine.

Kuhn et al., (1976) also found that morphine and pentazocine produce comparable discriminative effects in the rat. By log-probit analysis Kuhn et al., (1976) calculated that pentazocine was 0.4 times as potent as morphine as a discriminative stimulus which is in close accord with the potency ratio for these drugs estimated from the data of Shannon and Holtzman (1976a). The fact that rats trained with pentazocine as the discriminative stimulus generalize fully to morphine and vice versa is compelling evidence that the discriminative properties of the two drugs are very similar.

Six narcotic antagonists tested by Shannon and Holtzman (1976a, b) failed to substitute for the 3.0 mg/kg training dose of morphine insofar as they did not engender average levels of responding of at least 90% to the morphine-appropriate choice lever

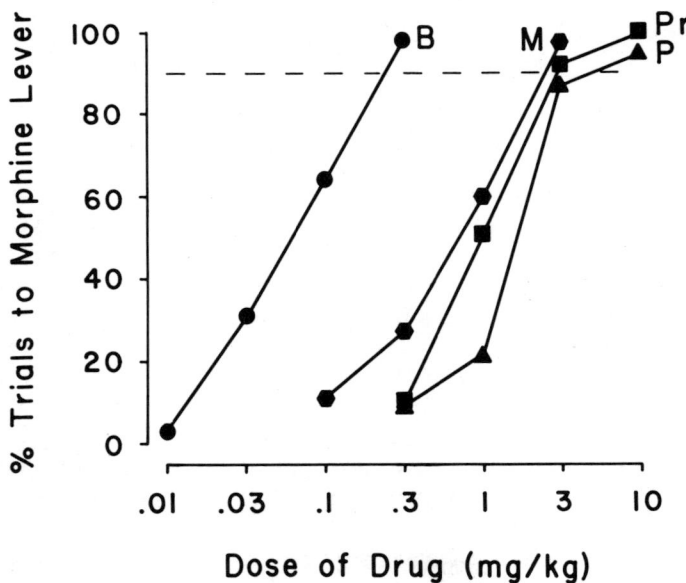

Figure 1. Morphine-like discriminative effects produced by morphine (M) and the narcotic antagonists butorphanol (B), profadol (Pr) and pentazocine (P) in rats trained to discriminate between saline and 3.0 mg/kg of morphine. Sessions consisted of 20 trials; the percentage of trials not completed on the morphine-appropriate choice lever were completed on the saline-appropriate lever. Each point is an average of one observation in each of 4-5 rats except for the morphine dose-response curve where each point represents an average based upon 20 rats. The dashed horizontal line indicates where 90% of the trials were completed on the morphine choice lever. After the administration of saline the animals consistently completed less than 10% of the trials on the morphine choice lever. Data are modified from Shannon and Holtzman (1976a, b).

TABLE 1. Narcotic antagonists that fail to produce discriminative effects equivalent to those of 3.0 mg/kg of morphine in the rat[a].

Drug	Dose Range Tested (mg/kg)[b]	Maximum Effect	
		Dose (mg/kg)	Percent Trials to Morphine Lever[c]
cyclazocine	0.03 - 3.0	0.3	83
nalbuphine	0.1 - 100	30	83
levallorphan	0.1 - 30	0.3	81
ketocyclazocine	0.3 - 3.0	1.0	71
Nalorphine	0.1 - 30	3.0	54
oxilorphan	0.3 - 30	1.0, 10	8

[a]Rats were trained to discriminate between saline and 3.0 mg/kg of morphine in a two-choice discrete trial avoidance procedure. Each session consisted of 20 trials. A drug was considered to produce discriminative effects equivalent to those produced by the training dose of morphine if the average number of trials completed by the group was at least 90% to the morphine-appropriate lever. An average of 98% of the trials were completed on the morphine-appropriate lever after the administration of 3.0 mg/kg of morphine, and 4.0% after the administration of saline. Data are modified from Shannon and Holtzman (1976a, b).

[b]Doses from each drug series were tested in a random sequence in 4-5 rats.

[c]Remaining trials were completed on the saline-appropriate choice lever.

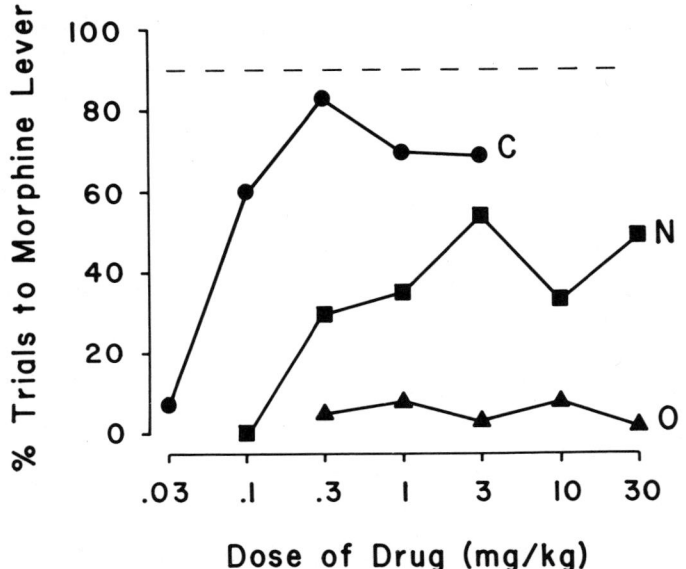

Figure 2. Failure of cyclazocine (C), nalorphine (N) and oxilorphan (O) to produce discriminative effects comparable to those of 3.0 mg/kg of morphine in rats trained to discriminate between saline and 3.0 mg/kg of morphine. Details are as in Fig. 1.

at any of the doses tested (Table 1). Dose-response curves
representative of this group of antagonists are presented in Fig.
2. The shallowness of the dose-response functions and the
appearance of a "ceiling" on the maximum percent trials completed on the morphine-appropriate choice lever stand in marked
contrast to the dose-response characteristics of the drugs shown
in Fig. 1. On the other hand, with the exception of oxilorphan,
narcotic antagonists that did not substitute for the morphine
training dose generally produced greater levels of responding on
the morphine-appropriate choice lever than did a variety of non-
opioid psychoactive drugs that were tested up to doses that produced signs of motor impairment in the rats (Table 2).

In spite of marked differences in experimental procedures,
the discriminative effects of cyclazocine (0.08 - 2.5 mg/kg),
nalorphine (10 - 160 mg/kg) and pentazocine (10 mg/kg) in the
study by Colpaert et al., (1976) were remarkably similar to those
reported by Shannon and Holtzman (1976a, b), particularly with
respect to the shape of the dose-response curves for cyclazocine
and nalorphine. The principal difference in findings between the
two studies resides in the slightly higher peak drug effects
obtained in the former. Thus, 100% of the animals responded on
the fentanyl-appropriate lever at 0.31 mg/kg of cyclazocine and
80% at 40 mg/kg of nalorphine (Colpaert et al., 1976). These
maximum drug effects can be compared with those presented in
Table 1.

Stimulus Generalization as a Function of Training Dose

It is not surprising that the stimulus generalization curves
for a given drug are shifted to the right or to the left along the
abscissa as the training dose of that same drug is increased or
decreased, respectively (Overton, 1974). However, the magnitude of the training dose acquires added significance when testing
for generalization to drugs that have a substantially lower efficacy
than the training dose (i.e., partial agonists) or which possess
multiple components of action where the contribution of any one
component to the pharmacological activity of the drug relative to
all other components may be a direct function of dose. Both of
these features are found among analgesics with mixed agonist
and antagonist properties. Accordingly, the magnitude of the
training dose must be carefully considered in any evaluation of the
discriminative effects of narcotic antagonists based upon generalization experiments in rats trained with a pure agonist such as
morphine. As an example, Shannon and Holtzman (unpublished
observations) found that the maximum number of trials completed
on the morphine-appropriate choice lever after the administration
of cyclazocine decreased from 83 to 23% when the training dose of

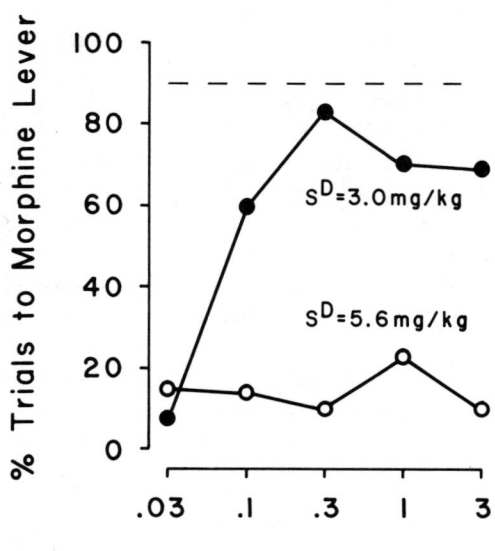

Figure 3. Discriminative effects of cyclazocine as a function of the training dose of morphine. Cyclazocine dose response curves were determined in two separate groups of rats: one trained to discriminate between saline and 3.0 mg/kg of morphine and the other trained to discriminate between saline and 5.6 mg/kg of morphine. Data are from Shannon and Holtzman (unpublished observations). Other details are as in Fig. 1.

TABLE 2. Absence of morphine-like discriminative effects with non-opioid psychoactive drugs in the rat[a]

Drug	Dose Range Tested (mg/kg)	Maximum Effect Dose (mg/kg)	Percent Trials to Morphine Lever
d-amphetamine	0.1 - 3.0	3.0	61
scopolamine	0.01 - 1.0	0.1	49
ketamine	1.0 - 30	10	34
pentobarbital	3.0 - 17.5	10	30
chlorpromazine	0.1 - 3.0	0.3	17
physostigmine	0.03 - 1.0	0.1	11
mescaline	3.0 - 100	10-100	3

[a]Details are as in Table 1.

morphine was increased from 3.0 to 5.6 mg/kg (Fig. 3). In contrast, the increase in training dose resulted in a one-half log-dose shift to the right of the dose-response curve for the partial morphine agonist profadol without any decrement in maximum effect (Fig. 4). This concept may afford an explanation of why rats trained with 0.04 mg/kg of fentanyl (Colpaert et al., 1976) or 3.0 mg/kg of morphine (Shannon and Holtzman, 1976b) show partial generalization to nalorphine whereas rats trained with 10 mg/kg of morphine (Gianutsos and Lal, 1976) show none.

Blockade of Discriminative Effects of Narcotic Antagonists

One of the features of a specific narcotic effect is that it can be reversed by specific narcotic antagonists (see Martin, 1967). The pure antagonist naloxone has been routinely used as a pharmacological tool for characterizing the discriminative properties of narcotic analgesics (e.g., Rosecrans et al., 1973; Winter, 1975; Shannon and Holtzman, 1976a,c). In addition to being an antagonist of the classical narcotic agonists, naloxone can block many of the actions of the mixed agonist-antagonists (Blumberg and Dayton, 1973), including discriminative effects.

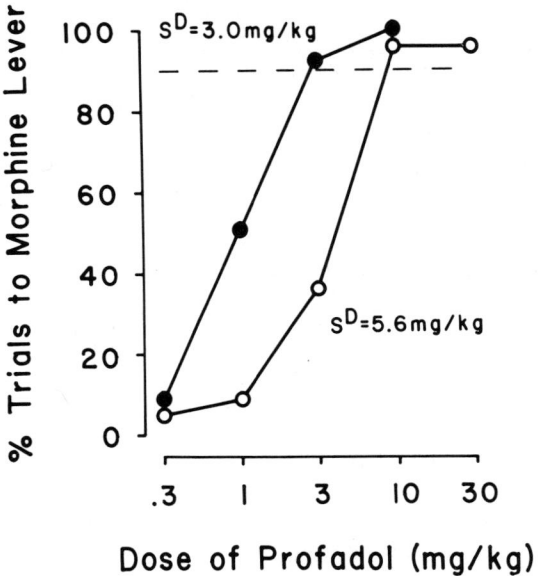

Figure 4. Discriminative effects of profadol as a function of the training dose of morphine. Details are as in Fig. 3.

Kuhn et al. (1976) found that 0.4 mg/kg of naloxone reduced the percent of responses on the pentazocine-appropriate choice lever from 81% to 41% after 10 mg/kg of pentazocine, and from 86% to 16% after 7.5 mg/kg of morphine. The greater sensitivity of the discriminative effects of morphine to antagonism by naloxone than the discriminative effects of pentazocine is consistent with other reports that naloxone is more potent in blocking the actions of pure agonists than in blocking the effects of drugs with mixed agonist and antagonist properties (Kosterlitz and Watt, 1968; Holtzman, 1976a). Naloxone itself (0.4 mg/kg) had no pentazocine-like discriminative effects, and has not been found to exhibit opiate-like discriminative effects even at doses in excess of 100 mg/kg (Colpaert et al., 1976).

IV. DISCRIMINATIVE PROPERTIES IN THE SQUIRREL MONKEY

Monkeys Trained with Morphine

Since studies on the discriminative effects of narcotic antagonists in primates are only now beginning to emerge in their early stages (Schaefer and Holtzman, 1976 and unpublished observations), they can be summarized with relative brevity. It is becoming apparent that many narcotic antagonists that completely or partially substituted for 3.0 mg/kg of morphine in rats trained to discriminate between morphine and saline do not show that same level of activity in squirrel monkeys also trained to discriminate between saline and 3.0 mg/kg of morphine (Table 3). In each instance the drugs were tested up to the highest dose compatible with maintaining the well-being of the animals. There are many possible interpretations of these results but two seem most plausible. The first is that the differences in results reflect true differences in the response of each species to the drugs being tested. For example, the squirrel monkey may be capable of distinguishing between morphine and pentazocine whereas the rat is not. The second possibility raises again the question of the magnitude of the training dose. Although both the rat and the squirrel monkey were trained with 3.0 mg/kg of morphine, this dose may be a more intense discriminative stimulus in the latter species than in the former. When 3.0 mg/kg of morphine was given to rats and squirrel monkeys lever pressing under a continuous shock avoidance schedule the response rate of the monkeys was depressed to a far greater extent than was the response rate of the rats (Holtzman, 1974, 1976b), and the ongoing behavior of squirrel monkeys performing under a schedule of food reinforcement was virtually eliminated by 3.0 mg/kg of morphine (Goldberg et al., 1976) whereas food-reinforced responding of rats showed little disruption after the same dose (Thompson et al., 1970). Thus, in terms of effects produced, 3.0 mg/kg of morphine

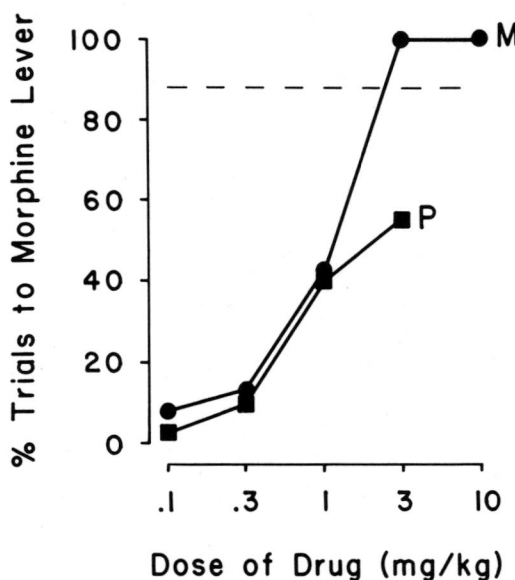

Figure 5. Comparison of the discriminative effects of morphine (M) and pentazocine (P) in squirrel monkeys trained to discriminate between saline and 3.0 mg/kg of morphine. Sessions consisted of 25 trials; the percentage of trials not completed on the morphine-appropriate choice lever were completed on the saline-appropriate lever. Each point is an average of one observation in each of 4 monkeys. The dashed horizontal line indicates where 88% of the trials were completed on the morphine choice lever. After the administration of saline the animals consistently completed less than 12% of the trials on the morphine choice lever. Data are modified from Schaefer and Holtzman (1976, and unpublished observations).

represents a relatively higher dose in the monkey than in the rat. In support of this interpretation is the fact that the maximum percentage of trials completed on the morphine-appropriate choice lever, following the administration of pentazocine, cyclazocine and nalbuphine occurred at the highest dose of those drugs that could be safely tested, and responding on the morphine-appropriate lever reached a plateau midway in the butorphanol dose-response curve (Table 3). With a training dose more comparable to the one used in the rat it is likely that some of these narcotic antagonists would have completely substituted for morphine. A comparison of the dose-response curves for morphine and pentazocine in the monkey is presented in Fig. 5.

Monkeys Trained with Cyclazocine

At the present time more narcotic antagonists have been tested in monkeys trained to discriminate vehicle from 0.1 mg/kg of cyclazocine (Schaefer and Holtzman, 1976) than have been tested in the monkeys trained on the saline vs. morphine discrimination. Monkeys trained with 0.1 mg/kg of cyclazocine generalized completely to ketocyclazocine (0.1 mg/kg), levallorphan (3.0 mg/kg) and oxilorphan. Morphine and the narcotic antagonists nalorphine, nalbuphine and pentazocine failed to substitute for the training dose of cyclazocine (Table 4, Fig. 6). Relatively few trials were completed on the cyclazocine-appropriate lever following the administration of psychoactive drugs from pharmacological classes unrelated to the narcotic agonists and antagonists (Table 5).

In antagonism experiments it was found that the discriminative effects of 0.1 mg/kg of cyclazocine were completely blocked by 1.0 mg/kg of naloxone; only 0.03 - 0.1 mg/kg of naloxone was necessary to block the discriminative effects of 3.0 mg/kg of morphine in the monkeys trained on the saline vs. morphine discrimination. However conclusions based upon comparisons of drug effects between the two groups of monkeys would be premature before the relative discriminability of the training drugs can be ascertained.

V. DISCRIMINATION AS AN ANIMAL MODEL OF SUBJECTIVE DRUG EFFECTS

In general, there appears to be a good correspondence between the discriminative effects of narcotic antagonists in infrahuman species and the subjective effects that these drugs produce in man. In the studies by Shannon and Holtzman (1976a, b), three narcotic antagonists which produce predominantly euphoric or morphine-like subjective effects in man - profadol, pentazocine

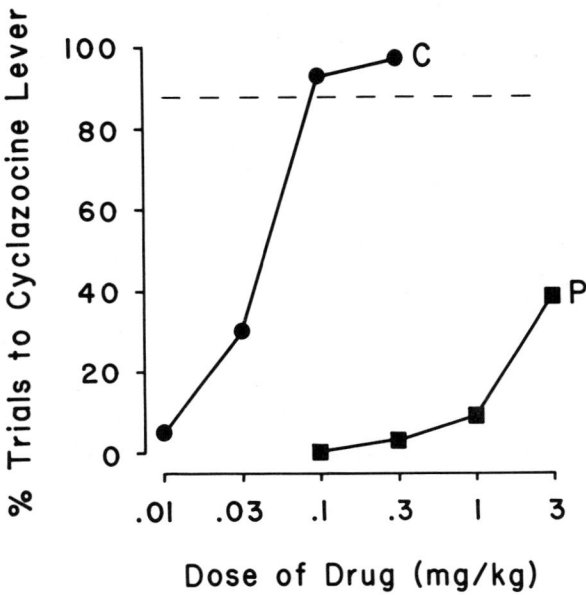

Figure 6. Comparison of the discriminative effects of cyclazocine (C) and pentazocine (P) in squirrel monkeys trained to discriminate between vehicle and 0.1 mg/kg of cyclazocine. Details are as in Fig. 5.

TABLE 3. Narcotic antagonists that fail to produce effects equivalent to those of 3.0 mg/kg of morphine in the monkey[a]

Drug	Dose Range Tested (mg/kg)[b]	Maximum Effect Dose (mg/kg)	% Trials to Morphine Lever[c]
butorphanol	0.003 - 3.0	0.1, 1.0	75
nalbuphine	1.0 - 30	30	64
cyclazocine	0.01 - 0.3	0.3	57
pentazocine	0.1 - 3.0	3.0	55

[a] Monkeys were trained to discriminate between saline and 3.0 mg/kg of morphine in a two-choice discrete trial avoidance procedure. Each session consisted of 25 trials. A drug was considered to produce discriminative effects equivalent to those produced by the training dose of morphine if the average number of trials completed by the group was at least 88% to the morphine-appropriate lever. An average of 100% of the trials were completed on the morphine-appropriate lever after the administration of 3.0 mg/kg of morphine, and 5% after the administration of saline. Data are modified from Schaefer and Holtzman (1976 and unpublished observations).

[b] Doses from each drug series were tested in a random sequence in 3-4 monkeys.

[c] Remaining trials were completed on the saline-appropriate choice lever.

and butorphanol (Jasinski et al., 1970, 1971, 1975) - also produced discriminative effects in the rat comparable to those produced by the training dose of morphine. The profile of subjective effects produced by nalmexone, a drug which also substituted for morphine in the rat, has not yet been described.

The results of experiments with antagonists of the cyclazocine type are also concordant with the reported subjective effects of these drugs in man. Cyclazocine, nalorphine, levallorphan and oxilorphan (Martin et al., 1965; Martin and Gorodetzky, 1965; Jasinski et al, 1967; Haertzen, 1970, 1974; Jasinski and Nutt, 1973) produce what Martin (1967) has termed a "nalorphine syndrome"

TABLE 4. Morphine and narcotic antagonists that fail to produce discriminative effects equivalent to those of 0.1 mg/kg of cyclazocine in the monkey[a]

Drug	Dose Range Tested (mg/kg)	Maximum Effect Dose (mg/kg)	% Trials to Cyclazocine Lever[b]
nalorphine	0.1 - 100	10	72
morphine	0.1 - 5.6	5.6	52
nalbuphine	1.0 - 30	10	39
pentazocine	0.1 - 3.0	3.0	39

[a] Monkeys were trained to discriminate between vehicle and 0.1 mg/kg of cyclazocine in a two-choice discrete trial avoidance procedure. An average of 93% of the trials were completed on the cyclazocine-appropriate lever after the administration of 0.1 mg/kg of cyclazocine, and 2% after the administration of vehicle. Other details are as in Table 3.

of dysphoria. The subjective effects of ketocyclazocine in man have not been reported but would be anticipated to be essentially similar to those of cyclazocine based upon the preclinical observation that ketocyclazocine produced a dose-related suppression of the cyclazocine abstinence syndrome in the cyclazocine-dependent chronic spinal dog (Gilbert and Martin, 1976). None of these drugs produced discriminative effects in the rat comparable to those of 3.0 mg/kg of morphine. Although rats trained with 0.04 mg/kg of fentanyl did completely generalize to one dose of cyclazocine (Colpaert et al., 1976), seemingly disparate findings between studies may be reconciled when data becomes available on the relative intensity of discriminative stimuli engendered by different training drugs.

Nalbuphine also failed to produce discriminative effects in the rat that were equivalent to the training dose of morphine. In man nalbuphine resembles pentazocine in that both possess a mixture of morphine-like and nalorphine-like properties (Jasinski and Mansky, 1972). However, the nalorphine-like component of action is more prominent in nalbuphine than it is in pentazocine.

Cyclazocine, nalorphine and levallorphan also have a morphine-like component of action in man which is especially evident

TABLE 5. Absence of cyclazocine-like discriminative effects with non-opioid psychoactive drugs in the monkey[a]

Drug	Dose Range Tested (mg/kg)	Maximum Effect Dose (mg/kg)	% Trials to Cyclazocine Lever[b]
scopolamine	0.01 - 0.3	0.1	41
mescaline	1.0 - 30	30	32
d-amphetamine	0.03 - 1.0	1.0	15
pentobarbital	1.0 - 5.6	5.6	1

[a] Details are as in Table 4.

at low doses and often results in these compounds being identified as "dope" or morphine in double-blind tests of single doses in postaddict volunteers (Martin and Gorodetzky, 1965; Martin et al., 1965; Haertzen, 1974). It is tempting to speculate that the relatively high level of morphine-appropriate responding following the administration of these drugs (Shannon and Holtzman, 1976a,b; Colpaert et al., 1976; also, see Table 1) is a reflection of their morphine-like component of action. Although there was no allusion to the presence or absence of morphine-like activity in the preliminary report of oxilorphan's subjective effects (Jasinski and Nutt, 1973), it has been postulated (Martin et al., 1976) that, at least in the dog, the agonist activity of oxilorphan is mediated by a population of receptors distinct from those which mediate the effects of morphine. This view is compatible with the finding that oxilorphan was not discriminably different from saline in rats trained to discriminate between saline and morphine (c.f., Fig. 2).

Direct assessment of the cyclazocine-like discriminative properties of narcotic antagonists in the monkey yielded data complementary with those obtained in the rat and in general accord with the known subjective effects produced by the drugs in man. However, the parallelism between the discriminative effects of narcotic antagonists in cyclazocine-trained monkeys and subjective effects was not perfect. Most notably, nalorphine, which produces subjective effects in man highly similar to those of cyclazocine (Martin et al., 1965; Haertzen, 1970), resulted in a maximum of only 72% of the trials being completed on the cyclazocine-appropriate lever. On the other hand, Martin et al., (1965) observed that the peak subjective effects of nalorphine were less intense than the peak effects of cyclazocine. Nalorphine also has a lower efficacy than cyclazocine for depressing the flexor reflex of the chronic spinal dog (McClane and Martin, 1967), producing analgesia in a modified hot-plate test in the rat (O'Callaghan and Holtzman, 1975), and suppressing the cyclazocine withdrawal syndrome in the cyclazocine-dependent dog (Gilbert and Martin, 1976). Thus, although nalorphine has long been regarded as the prototype of the analgesics with mixed agonist and narcotic-antagonist properties (e.g., Woods, 1956; Martin, 1967), this view probably stems more from nalorphine's chronology than from its pharmacology. The results of recent studies indicate that it would be more appropriate to view nalorphine as a partial cyclazocine agonist (Gilbert and Martin, 1976). When considered within this framework, the failure of cyclazocine-trained monkeys to generalize completely to the stimulus properties of nalorphine is not incongruous with the close similarity of the subjective effects that these drugs produce in man. Nevertheless, such a conclusion could not have been arrived at by viewing the data from the drug discrimination experiment in isolation from the existing body of literature on narcotic antagonists. As suggested by the results of studies in the rat, the use of multiple training doses would undoubtedly facilitate accurate evaluation of the discriminative properties of narcotic antagonists in the monkey.

Presently, data on the discriminative effects of pentazocine-type compounds in the monkey do not show the concordance with subjective effects in man that the data derived from experiments in the rat show. Neither pentazocine which is principally euphoric nor nalbuphine which is more dysphoric substituted for either the training dose of morphine or the training dose of cyclazocine. Monkeys trained on the saline vs. morphone discrimination generalized only partially to butorphanol which has prominent morphine-like activity in man (butorphanol was not tested in the monkeys trained with cyclazocine). Two possible explanations for these results have already been advanced (vida supra). One relates to species specificity; the discriminative stimuli produced by the pentazocine-type drugs in the squirrel monkey may be qualitatively different from those produced in the rat or in man. It is well know that the effects of morphine on behavior vary dramatically among species (see Krueger et al., 1941; Seevers and Deneau, 1963). The other explanation involves the magnitude of the training dose. High training doses would be inappropriate for detecting a component of drug action that has a substantially lower efficacy than that of the training drug.

There is also a third factor that requires consideration: the procedure for categorizing the subjective effects of narcotic antagonists in man. Typically, this is accomplished by administering a series of single doses to postaddict volunteers under double-blind conditions and recording their responses on a subjective drug-effect questionnaire made up of item groupings from the Addiction Research Center Inventory (Jasinski et al., 1968; Haertzen, 1970, 1974). The qualitative nature of a drug's subjective effects is determined on the basis of the scores produced by the drug in the various item groupings. Whereas in discrimination paradigms drugs are tested in animals trained to rigorous performance criteria with a reference compound such as morphine or cyclazocine, in the clinical situation drugs are compared with reference compounds indirectly via the subjective drug-effect questionnaires. Simply because two drugs produce similar scores on subjective questionnaires should not imply that the drugs would not be discriminable from each other if they were compared directly in the same subject. Accordingly, pentazocine-type narcotic antagonists might be discriminable from both cyclazocine and morphine if these drugs were compared more directly. Most probably, there is some element of merit to each of the possible explanations.

VI. CONCLUSIONS

Analgesics with mixed agonist and narcotic antagonist properties can produce several complex syndromes of subjective disturbances the qualitative nature of which is a principal determinant of the drugs' abuse potential. The results of studies described in this chapter suggest that drug discrimination paradigms may provide an animal model for the preclinical evaluation of this important component of action of the narcotic antagonists. However, a large number of experiments remain to be performed in order to develop this model to the point where it will yield reliable and readily interpretable data. Narcotic antagonists with actions representative of the broad spectrum of subjective effects obtainable in man should be tested in at least two animal species in which subgroups of subjects have been trained to discriminate saline from a standard narcotic agonist such as morphine or fentanyl and drug vehicle from cyclazocine. The use of other placebo-drug discriminations such as vehicle vs. pentazocine and drug-drug discriminations such as morphine vs. cyclazocine could also be advantageous. In each case, the intensity of the discriminative stimuli engendered by the training drugs must be defined. Moreover, test drugs should be evaluated in different groups of subjects which have been trained to discriminate different doses of the same drug. Finally, the ultimate validation of this type of animal model must evolve empirically. Toward this objective, there will have to be collaboration between the clinician and the basic scientist in order to resolve disparities which might arise between animal and clinical data.

VII. ACKNOWLEDGEMENTS

The research of the authors described in this chapter was supported in part by the following U.S. Public Health Service Grants: DA00541, 2T1 GM179 National Research Service Award DA 05020 to G.J.S. and Research Scientist Development Award K02 DA00008 to S.G.H.

VIII. REFERENCES

Archer, S. and Harris, L.S.: Narcotic antagonists. In Progress in Drug Research, ed. by E. Jucker, pp 261-320, Birkhauser Verlag, Basel, 1965.

Blumberg, H. and Dayton, H.B.: Naloxone and related compounds. In Agonist and Antagonist Actions of Narcotic Analgesic Drugs, ed. by H. W. Kosterlitz, H.O.J. Collier and J.E. Villarreal, pp. 110-119, University Park Press, Baltimore, 1973.

Colpaert, F.C., Niemegeers, C.J.E. and Janssen, P.A.: On the ability of narcotic antagonists to produce the narcotic cue. J. Pharmacol. Exp. Ther. 197: 180-187, 1976.

Fraser, H.F.: Methods for assessing the addiction liability of opioids and opioid antagonists in man. In the Addictive States, ed. by A. Wikler, pp. 176-187, Williams and Wilkins Co., Baltimore, 1968.

Gianutsos, G. and Lal, H.: Effect of loperamide, haloperidol and methadone in rats trained to discriminate morphine from saline. Psychopharmacologia 41: 267-270, 1975.

Gianutsos, G. and Lal, H.: Selective interaction of drugs with a discriminable stimulus associated with narcotic action. Life Sci. 19: 91-98, 1976.

Gilbert, P.E. and Martin, W.R.: The effects of morphine- and nalorphine-like drugs in the nondependent, morphine-dependent and cyclazocine-dependent chronic spinal dog. J. Pharmacol. Exp. Ther., 198: 66-82, 1976.

Goldberg, S.R., Morse, W.H. and Goldberg, D.M.: Some behavioral effects of morphine, naloxone and nalorphine in the squirrel monkey and pigeon. J. Pharmacol. Exp. Ther. 196: 625-636, 1976.

Haertzen, C.A.: Subjective effects of narcotic antagonists cyclazocine and nalorphine in the Addiction Research Center Inventory (ARCI) Psychopharmacologia 18: 366-377, 1970.

Haertzen, C.A.: Subjective effects of narcotic antagonists. In Narcotic Antagonists, ed. by M.C. Braude, L.S. Harris, E.L. May, J.P. Smith and J.E. Villarreal, pp. 383-398, Raven Press, New York, 1974.

Holtzman, S.G.: Tolerance to the stimulant effects of morphine and pentazocine on avoidance responding in the rat. Psychopharmacologia 39: 23-37, 1974.

Holtzman, S.G.: Comparison of the effects of morphine, pentazocine, cyclazocine and amphetamine on intracranial self-stimulation in the rat. Psychopharmacologia 46: 223-227, 1976a.

Holtzman, S.G.: Effects of morphine and narcotic antagonists on avoidance behavior of the squirrel monkey. J. Pharmacol. Exp. Ther. 196: 145-155, 1976b.

Isbell, H.: Attempted addiction to nalorphine. Fed. Proc. 15: 442, 1956.

Jasinski, D.R.: Effects in man of partial morphine agonists. In Agonist and Antagonist Actions of Narcotic Analgesic Drugs, ed. by H.W. Kosterlitz, H.O.J. Collier and J.E. Villarreal, pp. 94-103, University Park Press, Baltimore, 1973a.

Jasinski, D.R.: Narcotic antagonists as analgesics of low dependence liability - theoretical and practical implications of recent studies. In Yearbook of Drug Abuse, ed. by L. Brill and E. Harms, pp. 37-48, Behavioral Publications, New York, 1973b.

Jasinski, D.R., Griffith, J.D., Pevnick, J.S. and Clark, S.C.: Progress report on studies from the Clinical Pharmacology Section of the Addiction Research Center. Reported to the 37th Meeting of the Committee on Problems of Drug Dependence, 1975.

Jasinski, D.R. and Mansky, P.A.: Evaluation of nalbuphine for abuse potential. Clin. Pharmacol. Ther. 13: 78-90, 1972.

Jasinski, D.R., Martin, W.R. and Haertzen, C.A.: The human pharmacology and abuse potential of N-allylnoroxymorphone (naloxone). J. Pharmacol. Exp. Ther. 157: 420-426, 1967.

Jasinski, D.R., Martin. W.R. and Hoeldtke, R.D.: Effects of short- and long-term administration of pentazocine in man. Clin. Pharmacol. Ther. 11: 285-403, 1970.

Jasinski, D.R., Martin, W.R. and Hoeldtke, R.: Studies of the dependence-producing properties of GPA-1657, profadol, and propiram in man. Clin. Pharmacol. Ther. 12: 613-649, 1971.

Jasinski, D.R., Martin, W.R. and Sapira, J.D.: Antagonism of the subjective, behavioral, pupillary, and respiratory depressant effects of cyclazocine by naloxone. Clin. Pharmacol. Ther. 9: 215-222, 1968.

Jasinski, D.R. and Nutt, J.G.: Progress report on the clinical assessment program of the addiction research center. Reported to the 35th Meeting of the Committee on Problems of Drug Dependence, 1973.

Kosterlitz, H.W. and Watt, A.J.: Kinetic parameters of narcotic agonists and antagonists with particular reference to N-allylnoroxymorphone (naloxone). Brit. J. Pharmacol. 33: 266-276, 1968.

Krueger, H., Eddy, N.B. and Sumwalt, M.: The pharmacology of opium alkaloids. Publ. Hlth. Rep. 56 (Suppl. 165): Parts I and II, 1941.

Kuhn, D.M., Greenberg, I. and Appel, J.B.: Stimulus properties of the narcotic antagonist pentazocine: Similarity to morphine and antagonism by naloxone. J. Pharmacol. Exp. Ther. 196: 121-127, 1976.

Lasagna, L. and Beecher, H.K.: The analgesic effectiveness of nalorphine and nalorphine-morphine combinations in man. J. Pharmacol. Exp. Ther. 112: 356-363, 1954.

Lewis, J.W., Bentley, K.W. and Cowan, A.: Narcotic analgesics and antagonists. Annu. Rev. Pharmacol. 11: 241-270, 1971.

Martin, W.R.: Opioid antagonists. Pharmacol. Rev. 19: 463-521, 1967.

Martin, W. R. , Eades, C. G. , Thompson, J. A. , Huppler, R. E. and Gilbert, P. E. : The effects of morphine- and nalorphine-like drugs in the nondependent and morphine-dependent chronic spinal dog. J. Pharmacol. Exp. Ther. , in press, 1976.

Martin, W. R. , Fraser, H. F. , Gorodetzky, C. W. and Rosenberg, D. E. : Studies of the dependence-producing potential of the narcotic antagonist 2-cyclo-propylmethyl-2'-hydroxy-5, 9-dimethyl-6, 7-benzomorphan (cyclazocine, WIN-20, 740, ARC II-C-3). J. Pharmacol. Exp. Ther. 150: 426-436, 1965.

Martin, W. and Gorodetzky, C. W. : Demonstration of tolerance to and physical dependence on N-allynormorphone (nalorphine). J. Pharmacol. Exp. Ther. 150: 437-442, 1965.

McClane, T. K. and Martin, W. R. : Effects of morphine, nalorphine, cyclazocine, and naloxone on the flexor reflex. Int. J. Neuropharmacol. 6: 89-98, 1967.

O'Callaghan, J. P. and Holtzman, S. G. : Quantification of the analgesic activity of narcotic antagonists by a modified hot-plate procedure. J. Pharmacol. Exp. Ther. 192: 497-505, 1975.

Overton, D. A. : Experimental methods for the study of state-dependent learning. Fed. Proc. 33: 1800-1813, 1974.

Rosecrans, J. A. , Goodloe, M. H. , Bennett, G. J. and Hirschorn, I. D. : Morphine as a discriminative cue: Effects of amine depletors and naloxone. Europ. J. Pharmacol. 21: 252-256, 1973.

Schaefer, G. J. and Holtzman, S. G. : Discriminative effects of morphine and cyclazocine in the squirrel monkey. Reported to the 38th Meeting of the Committee on Problems of Drug Dependence, 1976.

Seevers, M. H. and Deneau, G. A. : Phsyiological aspects of tolerance and physical dependence. In Physiological Pharmacology, ed. by W. S. Root and F. G. Hofman, vol. 1, pp. 565-640, Academic Press, New York, 1963.

Shannon, H. E. and Holtzman, S. G. : Evaluation of the discriminative effects of morphine in the rat. J. Pharmacol. Exp. Ther. , 198: 54-65, 1976a.

Shannon, H. E. and Holtzman, S. G. : Further evaluation of the discriminative effects of morphine in the rat. J. Pharmacol. Exp. Ther., in press, 1976b.

Shannon, H.E. and Holtzman, S.G.: Blockade of the discriminative effects of morphine in the rat by naltrexone and naloxone. Psychopharmacology in press, 1976c.

Thompson, T., Trombley, J., Luke, D. and Lott, D.: Effects of morphine on behavior maintained by four simple food-reinforcement schedules. Psychopharmacologia 17: 182-192, 1970.

Villarreal, J.E.: The effects of morphine agonists and antagonists on morphine-dependent rhesus monkeys. In Agonist and Antagonist Actions of Narcotic Analgesic Drugs, ed. by H.W. Kosterlitz, H.O.J. Collier and J.E. Villarreal, pp. 73-93, University Park Press, Baltimore, 1973.

Villarreal, J.E.: Recent advances in the pharmacology of morphine-like drugs. In Drug Dependence, ed. by R.T. Harris, C.R. Schuster and D. McIsaac, pp. 83-116, University of Texas Press, Austin, 1970.

Winter, J.C.: The stimulus properties of morphine and ethanol. Psychopharmacologia 44: 209-214, 1975.

Woods, L.A.: The pharmacology of nalorphine (N-allylnormorphone). Pharmacol. Rev. 8: 175-198, 1956.

DISCRIMINABLE STIMULI PRODUCED
BY ALCOHOL AND OTHER CNS DEPRESSANTS

Herbert Barry, III and Edward C. Krimmer

Department of Pharmacology
University of Pittsburgh School of Pharmacy
Pittsburgh, PA 15261

I. INTRODUCTION

Discriminability from the nondrug condition constitutes a recently discovered attribute of drugs. One of the early findings (Overton, 1966) was that rats trained to discriminate pentobarbital from the nondrug condition chose the drug response in tests with several other sedative-hypnotic drugs (phenobarbital, ethyl alcohol, ethyl carbamate) and also with anti-anxiety agents (chlordiazepoxide, meprobamate). This indicated similarity among these drugs with respect to stimulus attributes.

Further experiments have indicated the existence of differential stimulus attributes of these drugs. Animals trained to discriminate chlordiazepoxide from the nondrug condition do not consistently choose the drug response in tests with pentobarbital (Overton, 1966); animals trained to discriminate pentobarbital from the nondrug condition do not consistently choose the drug response in tests with alcohol (Krimmer, 1974b). The present chapter summarizes these and further findings, including two experiments in which rats were trained to discriminate alcohol from pentobarbital. Tests with several doses of these drugs demonstrate a qualitative and not merely quantitative difference between these drugs with respect to stimulus attributes. A new model portrays the relationship between two dimensions of emotional response, to account for the attributes of similarity and difference between alcohol and pentobarbital. The model also shows the relative positions of several other drugs (chlorpromazine, pentylenetetrazol, bemegride, and amphetamine).

Although pentobarbital has been used as the prototype in much of the research on discriminable drug stimuli, alcohol has features of special interest and is emphasized in the present chapter. A high degree of generality of the alcohol stimulus is suggested by the consistent choice of the alcohol response in tests with other hypnotic-sedatives and with anti-anxiety agents. The frequent consumption of alcoholic beverages in many human societies suggests that the effects of alcohol may have special attraction or benefit for many people. This might be related to the discriminative stimulus attributes of this drug.

II. ATTRIBUTES OF DISCRIMINABLE DRUG STIMULUS

The discriminable drug stimulus has been demonstrated by associating differential drug conditions with instrumental learning of alternative responses that alleviate an aversive unconditional stimulus. For example, animals may learn to press alternative levers that relieve hunger by obtaining a food pellet or that relieve pain by terminating shock to the grid floor. The instrumental responses thus become established as unconditional responses to the hunger or pain. The food reward or escape from shock becomes a subsequent unconditional stimulus.

The drug effect functions as a differential conditional stimulus or signal. Repeated pairings of alternative drug conditions with alternative unconditional responses, such as pressing different levers, cause the responses to become conditional responses, associated with the conditional drug stimuli. This is the process of classical conditioning, described by Pavlov (1927). The conditional responses are maintained by their association with the reinforcing unconditional stimulus, such as food reward or escape from shock. This is the association previously established by instrumental learning.

Strong unconditional stimulus effects of drugs are indicated by reinforcing and aversive effects of the drugs. These effects are demonstrated by animals that learn to self-administer a drug (Kelleher, 1976) or to avoid conditional stimuli associated with administration of a drug (Garcia, Hankins, Robinson and Vogt, 1972). When a drug functions as a discriminative signal, such unconditional stimulus effects must be subordinated to the different unconditional stimulus, such as food reward or shock escape, with which the drug effect is associated.

The usual sensory stimuli, such as visual or auditory signals, have been described as weak unconditional stimuli but distinctive conditional stimuli (Dollard and Miller, 1950). When drug conditions function as differential signals, it seems probable that the differential responses are based on distinctive rather than strong reinforcing or aversive effects of the drugs. Contrary to sensory signals, the drug effect usuallly has a delayed onset and changes slowly. The discrimination between drug and control conditions is generally trained at five minutes or longer after administration of the drug or control substance. Most sensory signals would be ineffective if such a long interval elapsed between their onset or other change and presentation of the opportunity for the differential responses. The pervasiveness and stability of the effects caused by drugs apparently compensate adequately for the disadvantageous long interval between drug administration and training.

III. DISCRIMINATION BETWEEN DRUG AND NONDRUG CONDITIONS

The initial demonstration of discrimination between alcohol and the control condition was one of a series of experiments by Conger (1951). The principal purpose was to demonstrate that alcohol diminishes shock avoidance more than food approach. Hungry rats were trained to run down a straight alley to obtain food. On each day when painful shock was delivered at the food cup, one group was administered alcohol (1200 mg/kg, intraperitoneally, 5 minutes earlier) and another group was administered the same volume of water (15 ml/kg). Avoidance of the food cup was learned less rapidly by the group for which alcohol was associated with the shock. This difference gave evidence that the avoidance response was more compatible with the nondrug than alcohol condition. The fact that both groups learned the differential response, measured by approach to the food cup on the first trial of the day, demonstrated that alcohol was an effective conditional stimulus for discrimination learning.

With the same dose, interval, and route, Barry, Koepfer and Lutch (1965) trained rats to turn in opposite directions in a T-maze for food pellets, under the differential conditions of alcohol and saline. Painful shocks and differential approach and avoidance responses were thereby shown to be unnecessary for the discrimination learning. Overton (1966) trained rats to turn in opposite directions in a T-maze to escape painful shock delivered to the grid floor, at 15 minutes after the differential treatments of a high alcohol dose (2400 mg/kg, intraperitoneally) or no injection. This was part of a series of experiments with similar procedures, mostly on barbiturates and antimuscarinic agents (Overton, 1962). Animals trained to discriminate alcohol from no treatment made the drug response in tests with pentobarbital (20 mg/kg), phenobarbital (80 mg/kg), ethyl carbamate (750 mg/kg), and meprobamate (200 mg/kg). Likewise, tests with alcohol elicited the drug response in animals trained to discriminate the same doses of these other drugs from saline (pentobarbital, phenobarbital) or from no treatment (ethyl carbamate, meprobamate).

Barry (1968) used a lever-pressing task to demonstrate that the discrimination between alcohol (1200 mg/kg) and saline, 5 minutes after intraperitoneal injection, did not depend on different motor responses or spatial locations associated with the differential

conditions. The rats were trained to maintain the illumination of
the test chamber in opposite conditions (on or off) depending on
whether they had been injected with alcohol or saline. Each lever
press reversed the illumination condition, and a food pellet was
delivered after accumulation of 20 seconds in the animal's correct
illumination condition for the alcohol or saline injection.
Successful learning by the rats to select the correct illumination
condition at the beginning of the session demonstrated that the
animals had learned a discriminative choice rather than separate,
dissociated habits associated with the alcohol and saline conditions.

In addition to the discriminative stimulus attribute of the
alcohol injection, a disinhibitory effect was indicated by the
further finding that the first lever press was made sooner after the
beginning of the session when the animals had been injected with
alcohol rather than saline (Barry, 1968). No differences were found
between the two injection substances in other measures of performance,
such as number of lever presses and percentage of time the
illumination was maintained in the correct condition.

Kubena and Barry (1969a; 1969b) compared two procedures for
training rats to discriminate between alcohol (1200 mg/kg) and saline,
injected intraperitoneally 5 minutes before the start of the test.
The animals were trained to obtain food pellets by pressing a lever in
a test chamber. One procedure was to deliver a food pellet after the
first press on one of two levers, depending on the substance injected,
after a variable interval averaging one minute since delivery of the
prior food pellet. This choice between two equivalent responses
resembled the procedures used by Overton (1962; 1966) and Barry,
Koepfer and Lutch (1965). The other procedure was to deliver either
a food pellet or painful electric shock, depending on the substance
injected, after each fifth press on a single lever. The opposite
approach and avoidance responses resembled the procedure used by
Conger (1951).

The animals trained with both procedures learned the
discrimination between the effects of the alcohol and saline
injections. Kubena and Barry (1969a) discussed the relative
advantages of the two procedures. Kubena and Barry (1969b) reported
that the drug response was selected after sufficiently high doses of
pentobarbital and chlordiazepoxide, tested with both procedures, and
chloral hydrate, tested only with the choice procedure. The saline
response was selected in tests with other drugs, including
chlorpromazine and d-amphetamine. In the conflict procedure, Barry
and Kubena (1972) reported a weak disinhibitory or fear-reducing
drug effect, indicated by a slight preponderance of approach over
avoidance responses, in a test with a low alcohol dose (300 mg/kg).
Larger effects of this type, however, were found in tests with low
doses of chlordiazepoxide (5 mg/kg) and pentobarbital (5 mg/kg).

The conflict procedure (Kubena and Barry, 1969a) was used by
Barry and Krimmer (1972) for training rats to discriminate
pentobarbital (10 mg/kg) from saline, at the longer interval of
15 minutes after intraperitoneal injection. The drug response was

selected in tests with sufficiently high doses of chlordiazepoxide, amobarbital, meprobamate, and chloral hydrate. Low doses of these drugs, and also low doses of pentobarbital, elicited preponderantly approach responses. The saline response was selected in tests with alcohol and chlorpromazine, and these drugs elicited preponderantly avoidance responses. This study gave the first indication of a difference between alcohol and pentobarbital with respect to discriminative stimulus attributes.

The choice procedure (Kubena and Barry, 1969a) was modified to deliver a food pellet the first time the animal pressed the correct lever after a fixed interval of 10 seconds since the prior delivery of a pellet. Krimmer (1974b) reported that rats trained to discriminate alcohol (1000 mg/kg) from saline, at an interval of 20 minutes after intraperitoneal injection, preponderantly selected the drug response in tests with sufficiently high doses of pentobarbital, chlordiazepoxide, diazepam, paraldehyde, and chloral hydrate. A preponderance of drug responses in tests after oral administration of alcohol (1500 mg/kg) or pentobarbital (15 mg/kg) demonstrated that the discrimination was based on the systemic drug effects rather than on perception of a local reaction at the site of injection.

A group of rats concurrently trained to discriminate pentobarbital (10 mg/kg) from saline selected the drug response in tests with sufficiently high doses of chlordiazepoxide, diazepam, and paraldehyde, but they selected the saline response in tests with alcohol and chloral hydrate. In accordance with these results, they selected the drug response in a test after oral administration of pentobarbital (15 mg/kg) and the saline response in a test after oral administration of alcohol (1500 mg/kg).

The same choice procedure was used to train rats to discriminate a high dose of chlordiazepoxide (20 mg/kg) from saline at 60 minutes after administration (Krimmer and Barry, unpublished data). Separate subgroups were trained with the intraperitoneal and oral routes of administration. The dru' response was elicited only partially in tests at 20 minutes after pentobarbital administration, and the saline response was preponderant in tests at 20 minutes after alcohol administration. These results are consistent with a report by Overton (1966), using opposite directions of shock escape in the T-maze, that rats trained to discriminate a high chlordiazepoxide dose (30 mg/kg) from no injection did not dependably make the drug response in a test with pentobarbital, although rats trained to discriminate pentobarbital (10 mg/kg) from no injection made the drug response in a test with chlordiazepoxide.

Bueno, Carlini, Finkelfarb and Suzuki (1976) trained rats to turn in opposite directions in a T-maze for food, depending on whether they had been injected intraperitoneally with alcohol (1200 mg/kg) or saline 5 minutes earlier. The alcohol response was selected in tests with a sufficiently high dose of pentobarbital.

Krimmer and Barry (1973a) and Krimmer (1974b) reported on a procedure for training rats to press alternative levers to escape painful shock, depending on which alternative substance had been administered prior to the session. The discrimination at 20 minutes after intraperitoneal injection was learned more slowly between alcohol (1000 mg/kg) and saline than by a separate group between pentobarbital (10 mg/kg) and saline. Krimmer (1974b) reported on tests with various drugs in two additional groups of rats trained by similar procedures to discriminate pentobarbital (10 mg/kg) from saline. The drug response was elicited by sufficiently high doses of alcohol, chlordiazepoxide, diazepam, and paraldehyde. Krimmer (1974b) also reported on another group trained by similar procedures to discriminate chlordiazepoxide (10 mg/kg) from saline, 30 minutes after intraperitoneal injection. The drug response was elicited by sufficiently high doses of diazepam, pentobarbital, and chlorpromazine. Subsequent, unpublished data showed that the drug response was also elicited by a sufficiently high dose of alcohol, but a further study indicated that alcohol elicited the drug response in animals trained to discriminate a higher dose of chlordiazepoxide (20 mg/kg) from saline at 60 minutes after injection in animals trained with the oral but not intraperitoneal route. Since the oral route gave evidence for weaker effects, this finding indicated that training with a higher chlordiazepoxide dose results in poorer generalization to the alcohol condition.

Table 1 summarizes estimates of the minimal effective dose (ED_{50}), eliciting 50% drug response, in four groups of rats trained to discriminate alcohol from saline. A simplified method specified by Barry (1974) was used for calculating the ED_{50} if it was not stated in the cited report. The discriminative response is a fairly sensitive measure of the effects of the three drugs shown, because the minimal effective doses are generally somewhat below those that strongly alter other types of behavior.

The ED_{50} for the discriminative effect might depend on the dose used for training. Therefore, a more valid test is to attempt to train the discrimination at lower doses than those shown in Table 1 (1000 or 1200 mg/kg). Overton (1972) presented data on the number of training sessions required for rats to learn the discrimination betwen alcohol, 20 minutes after intraperitoneal injection, and no treatment, in rats trained to escape shock by running in alternative directions in a T-maze. The average number of sessions was very large with doses below 1000 mg/kg and decreased progressively with increasing doses. Fewer than five sessions were required to the beginning of the criterion for learning (8 correct choices in 10 sessions) with doses of 2000-3000 mg/kg. These data indicate that in the studies summarized in Table 1, the doses used for training (1000-1200 mg/kg) were close to the minimum at which the discrimination can be learned fairly easily.

Under some conditions, however, the discrimination can be learned with lower doses. Winter (1975) trained rats to press a lever for food, which was delivered only after one of the alternative substances (630 mg/kg alcohol or saline) was injected intraperitoneally

Table 1

The ED_{50} doses in mg/kg for alcohol (Alc.), pentobarbital (Pent.), and chlordiazepoxide (CDP) are compared in groups of rats trained to discriminate the designated dose of alcohol from saline by the procedures specified.

Alcohol dose (mg/kg)	Interval (minutes)	Procedure; incentive	Reference	ED_{50} (mg/kg) in tests		
				Alc.	Pent.	CDP
1200	5	Single lever food-shock	Kubena & Barry (1969b)	528	5.0	6.3
1200	5	Two levers food	Kubena & Barry (1969b)	604	7.0	4.5
1000	20	Two levers food	Krimmer (1974b)	610	5.4	2.9
1200	5	T-maze food	Bueno et al. (1976)	479	12.3	Not tested

20 minutes earlier. The discriminative response consisted of differential rates of pressing a lever at the beginning of the session. Ando (1975), with a similar procedure, trained rats to discriminate a much lower dose of alcohol (100 mg/kg) from saline at 5 minutes after intravenous infusion through a chronically implanted catheter.

Intravenous infusion was used by Krimmer and Barry (1976) to train rats to discriminate pentobarbital (5 mg/kg) from saline at the much shorter interval of 15 seconds. The discriminative response consisted of active or passive shock avoidance in a two-compartment box. The ED_{50} for the drug response was 3.0 mg/kg in tests with pentobarbital, 1.6 mg/kg with chlordiazepoxide, and 348 mg/kg with alcohol. These values are all smaller than those in Table 1 at longer intervals after intraperitoneal injection. Some of the animals were subsequently trained to discriminate a higher dose of pentobarbital (10 mg/kg) from saline at 10 minutes after intraperitoneal injection. The drug response was elicited in tests with sufficiently high doses of pentobarbital (ED_{50} = 3.5 mg/kg) and chlordiazepoxide (ED_{50} = 2.5 mg/kg) but not alcohol.

Discrimination betwen alcohol and saline has been trained at a wide range of intervals after intraperitoneal injection, ranging from 5 to 20 minutes, shown in Table 1 and reported in the additional studies that have been reviewed. This effective time span agrees well with data presented by Overton (1972) on the number of training sessions required for rats to learn the discrimination between alcohol (2000 mg/kg, injected intraperitoneally) and no treatment, measured by alternative directions of escape from shock in a T-maze. Fewer than five sessions to the start of the criterion were required at all intervals betwen 5 and 30 minutes. The minimum number, at 10 minutes, was less than 3. Krimmer (1974b) reported that in rats trained to discriminate alcohol (1000 mg/kg) from saline by pressing alternative levers for food, at 20 minutes after intraperitoneal injection, the drug response was consistently selected at short intervals of 2.5 and 5 minutes after alcohol (1000 mg/kg). Also, in comparison with the usual 20-minute interval a lower dose was sufficient to elicit the drug response in a test at 5 minutes. The onset of the discriminative drug effect is evidently very rapid, and it persists more than 60 minutes after injection.

IV. DISCRIMINATION BETWEEN ALCOHOL AND PENTOBARBITAL

Some of the findings reviewed in the preceding section give strong evidence for differences between alcohol and pentobarbital with respect to their discriminative effects. The most direct and convincing demonstration of such differences, however, is to train animals to discriminate between the effects of the two drugs.

In an experiment summarized by Krimmer and Barry (1973b) and described in detail by Krimmer (1974b), eight rats were trained to press alternative levers for food, depending on whether they had been injected intraperitoneally with alcohol (1000 mg/kg) or pentobarbital (10 mg/kg) 20 minutes earlier. The six-minute training sessions began with a variable interval, ranging from zero to 60 seconds, during which no food was delivered. During the remainder of the sessions, a food pellet was delivered by the first press on the correct lever after an interval of 10 seconds or longer since the prior delivery of a pellet.

After 57 training sessions, divided between the two drugs, all eight animals were making a majority of lever presses on the correct lever during the initial portion of the session without food rewards. Interspersed among the 115 subsequent training sessions were 103 test sessions of 60 seconds under novel conditions without food reward. Figure 1 shows the percentage of presses on the alcohol lever during tests with various time intervals and doses, calculated separately for each rat and averaged for all the rats that made any responses on either lever. The values under the training conditions, coinciding with the dashed vertical lines, constitute the average for the training sessions with the maximum 60-second initial portion prior to the delivery of the first food pellet.

The upper graph of Figure 1 shows that the alcohol response was predominant at all the time intervals tested (2.5 - 120 minutes) after injection of alcohol with the dose of 1000 mg/kg used in the training sessions at the 20-minute interval. Injection of pentobarbital with the dose used in the training sessions (10 mg/kg) resulted in a preponderance of pentobarbital responses only at the shorter time intervals tested (2.5 - 40 minutes). This combination of results indicates that at these doses pentobarbital was a more distinctive signal, whereas the alcohol effect was more similar to the nondrug condition. Therefore the alcohol response was made after injection of either drug when the interval was so long that the drug effect was weak. The differential drug effect showed a rapid onset, within 2.5 minutes, and was stable, without any large or sudden changes throughout the intervals from 2.5 to 40 minutes.

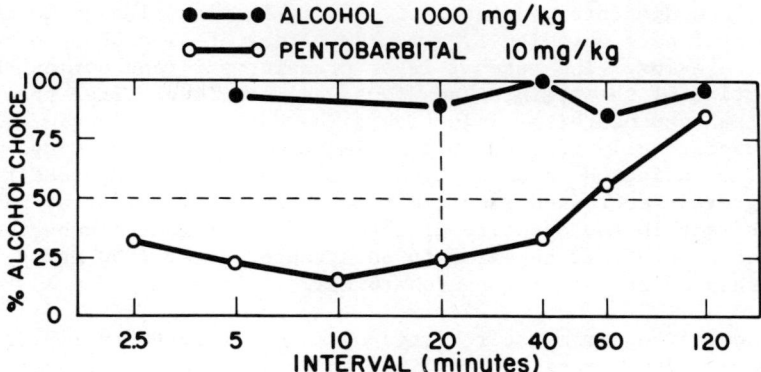

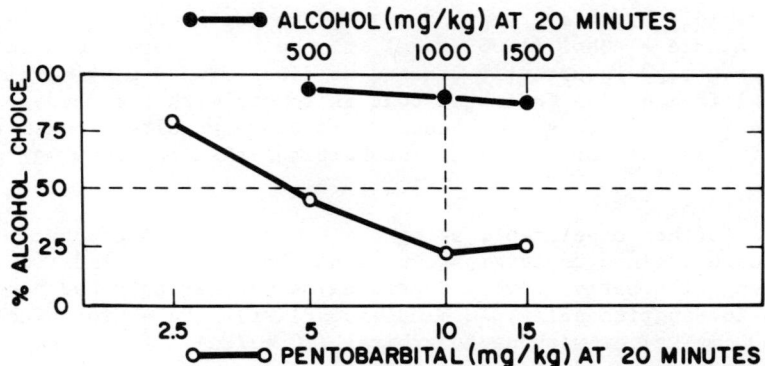

Figure 1. Percentage alcohol choice by eight rats trained to obtain food by pressing different levers at 20 minutes after intraperitoneal injection of alcohol (1000 mg/kg) or pentobarbital (10 mg/kg). The upper panel shows tests at several time intervals after these doses. The lower panel shows tests at 20 minutes after several doses.

The lower graph of Figure 1 shows the effects of different doses of alcohol (identified above the graph) and of pentobarbital (identified below the graph), tested at the 20-minute interval. The gradual change from pentobarbital to alcohol responses, after decreasing doses of pentobarbital, indicates that this drug was a more distinctive signal. Further evidence for this was a test at 20 minutes after saline injection, which resulted in 80% alcohol response. On the other hand, the persistence of the differential responses at the highest dose of both drugs indicates the presence of a qualitative and not merely quantitative difference between the effects of the two drugs. If alcohol had been a weaker signal of the same type as pentobarbital, the animals would have shifted to the pentobarbital response in the test after the highest alcohol dose.

The less distinctive signal of 1000 mg/kg alcohol than 10 mg/kg pentobarbital does not signify a weaker effect of alcohol on other types of behavior. The rate of lever pressing for food during the later portion of the training sessions was much lower after the alcohol than pentobarbital injection. The data from groups of animals concurrently trained to discriminate one of these drugs from saline indicated that in comparison with the nondrug condition, alcohol greatly decreased response rate whereas pentobarbital had a smaller effect in the opposite direction. Therefore the behaviorally depressant drug effect appeared to be stronger after 1000 mg/kg alcohol than after 10 mg/kg pentobarbital.

In another experiment, reported by Krimmer and Barry (1973a) and by Krimmer (1974b), rats were trained to escape shock by pressing alternative levers depending on whether they had been injected intraperitoneally with alcohol (1000 mg/kg) or pentobarbital (10 mg/kg) 20 minutes earlier. The discrimination was learned equally rapidly by this group and by a group concurrently trained to discriminate alcohol (1000 mg/kg) from saline. More rapid learning by another group concurrently trained to discriminate pentobarbital (10 mg/kg) from saline indicated that in common with the food-reward procedure (Fig. 1), this shock-escape procedure resulted in a more distinctive effect for 10 mg/kg pentobarbital than for 1000 mg/kg alcohol.

In a further experiment, using the shock-escape procedure, 12 rats were trained to terminate painful shock to the grid floor by pressing alternative levers depending on whether they had been injected intraperitoneally, 20 minutes earlier, with a high alcohol dose (1500 mg/kg) or with pentobarbital (10 mg/kg). The first 50 training sessions consisted of ten trials, each spaced one minute apart. After 50 sessions, divided between the two drugs, 43 test sessions under novel conditions were interspersed among 48 further training sessions of five trials each. Each test session consisted of a single trial in which the first press on either lever turned off the shock. The discriminative performance in the training sessions was measured by the first lever pressed on the first trial.

Figure 2 shows the results of some tests in six of the animals, selected on the basis of good discriminative performance during training sessions. Among the six rats excluded because of inferior discriminative performance, four failed to survive throughout the long series of tests. In the training sessions, which coincide with the vertical dashed lines, the percentage alcohol choice was much lower after 1500 mg/kg alcohol (Fig. 2) than after 1000 mg/kg alcohol (Fig. 1). This difference is probably due to the disadvantage of a smaller difference between the higher alcohol dose and pentobarbital (Fig. 2) with respect to distinctiveness of the signal. An alternative possibility is the strong, generalized depressant effect of the higher alcohol dose, thereby impairing performance of the discriminative response.

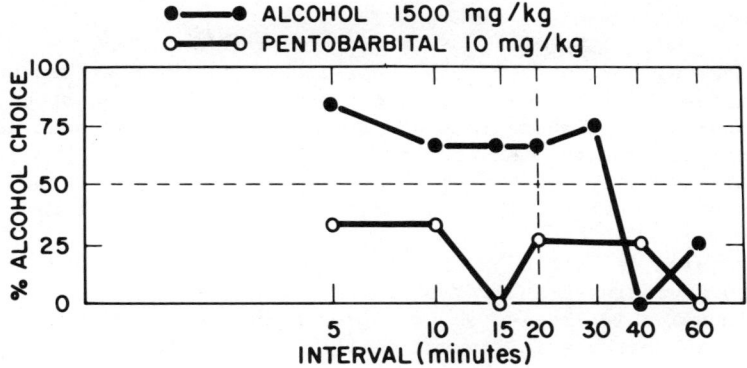
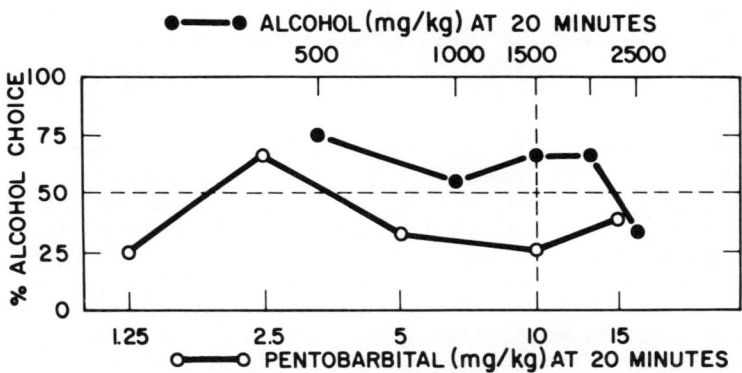

Figure 2. Percentage alcohol choice by six rats, with similar procedures and portrayals as in Figure 1 except that the animals were trained to escape shock instead of obtain food, and the alcohol dose was 1500 instead of 1000 mg/kg.

The lower graph of Figure 2 shows that for both drugs most of the doses tested, at the 20-minute interval, continued to elicit a preponderance of the choices learned in the training sessions. The alcohol response continued to be preponderant at a dose as low as 500 mg/kg, one-third of the dose of 1500 mg/kg used in training (identified above the graph). A sufficiently low alcohol dose would probably have resulted in a preponderance of pentobarbital responses, because a test at 20 minutes after saline injection elicited 40% alcohol response. The high alcohol dose of 2000 mg/kg continued to elicit a preponderance of alcohol responses. The deviant result in the test with 2500 mg/kg may be attributable to the almost anesthetic effect of this extremely high dose. The five pentobarbital doses, identified below the graph, elicited a preponderance of pentobarbital responses except for one deviant result with 2.5 mg/kg. If alcohol had been a stronger signal of the same type as pentobarbital, the animals would have shifted to the alcohol response in the test after the highest pentobarbital dose.

V. MODEL FOR RELATIONSHIPS AMONG DRUGS

The preceding portions of this chapter have reviewed evidence for similarities and also for differences among sedative-hypnotics, such as alcohol and pentobarbital, and anti-anxiety agents, such as chlordiazepoxide. Figure 3 shows a model that accounts for this mixture of similarities and differences in discriminative effects on the basis of dimensions of change from the nondrug condition.

One dimension is labeled as an increase in sedation in one direction and an increase in tension in the opposite direction. The other dimension is labeled as an increase in passivity in one direction and an increase in arousal in the opposite direction. The two dimensions are not orthogonal but instead are related to each other, so that sedation is closer to passivity than to arousal, and conversely tension is closer to arousal than to passivity. As a result of these relationships, the normal range shows more variation in the combined dimensions of sedation-passivity and tension-arousal than in the alternative combined dimensions of sedation-arousal and tension-passivity.

According to this model, alcohol primarily increases sedation, with a slight increase in passivity. Pentobarbital increases sedation and arousal to an equal degree. Chlordiazepoxide increases sedation, and its lack of a consistent effect on passivity or arousal places it intermediate between alcohol and pentobarbital. These differences are consistent with the effects of these drugs on other types of behavior. Wallgren and Barry (1970) characterized alcohol as producing more generalized depression of performance whereas pentobarbtial caused a greater degree of behavioral arousal due to stronger disinhibitory effects.

Another type of difference among these drugs is the degree of distinctiveness of the discriminative signal at a moderate dose, portrayed by the length of the line. Chlordiazepoxide is the most distinctive signal according to this model. Pentobarbital is more distinctive than alcohol, partly because of the small normal range for an equal combination of sedation and arousal.

A reasonable assumption is that the discriminative response transfers more readily to a more distinctive than to a less distinctive signal of the same type. Therefore, animals trained to discriminate a drug from saline would be more likely to choose the drug response in a test with a partially similar drug that is more distinctive rather than less distinctive. This accounts for the consistent choice of the alcohol response in tests with pentobarbital and chlordiazepoxide, in the studies summarized in Table 1 and also in the earlier study by Overton (1966). According to the model (Fig. 3), the discriminative alcohol signal is based almost entirely on the sedative effect, which deviates only slightly from the normal range. Pentobarbital and chlordiazepoxide both show larger deviations from the normal range in this respect.

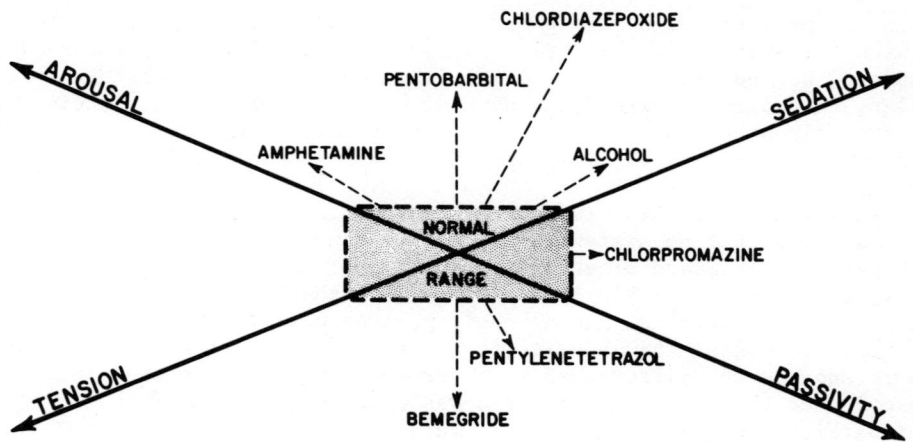

Figure 3. Model to account for similarities and differences among some sedative-hypnotic agents and related drugs with respect to their discriminative effects. The changes caused by each drug are located in terms of two dimensions: sedation-tension and arousal-passivity. The distance from the normal range, traversed by the arrow denoting each drug, portrays the degree to which a behaviorally moderate dose functions as a discriminative stimulus.

The effect of pentobarbital on sedation resembles alcohol but the effect of pentobarbital on arousal differs from alcohol. Barry and Krimmer (1972) and Krimmer (1974b) found that in two different lever-pressing tasks that involved food reward, rats trained to discriminate pentobarbital from saline did not select the drug response in tests with alcohol. This finding is explainable by this model if the food reward emphasizes the increase in arousal caused by pentobarbital or alternatively emphasizes the increase in passivity caused by alcohol. Krimmer (1974b) found that two separate groups of rats trained to discriminate pentobarbital from saline by a lever-pressing shock-escape response selected the drug response in tests with sufficiently high doses of alcohol. This is explainable by the model if shock emphasizes the increase in sedation caused by both drugs or alternatively shifts the effect of alcohol from passivity to arousal.

The model is consistent with the findings that animals trained to discriminate pentobarbital or alcohol from saline select the drug response in tests with chlordiazepoxide, even at low doses. The ED_{50} is lower for chlordiazepoxide than for pentobarbital in two of three studies summarized in Table 1, in two studies reviewed by Barry (1974), and in each of four experiments reported by Krimmer (1974b), in which rats were trained to discriminate alcohol or pentobarbital from saline. This generally greater distinctiveness of the chlordiazepoxide effect may be contrasted with the difference between these drugs in the doses required for incapacitating effects. Colpaert, Desmedt and Janssen (1976) found that loss of righting reflex, tested in rats at 30 minutes after intraperitoneal injection, required almost a ten-fold higher dose of chlordiazepoxide (204 mg/kg) than of pentobarbital (21.3 mg/kg).

Rats trained to discriminate a high chlordiazepoxide dose from saline do not consistently choose the drug response in tests with pentobarbital and alcohol (Overton, 1966; Krimmer and Barry, unpublished). This is explainable by the less distinctive effects of pentobarbital and alcohol, portrayed in Figure 3. One of the implications of the model is that higher doses of the drugs should enhance the differences among drugs. This is consistent with the evidence that the drug response was elicited by alcohol and pentobarbital to a lesser degree in rats trained to discriminate 20 mg/kg chlordiazepoxide from saline (Krimmer and Barry, unpublished) than in rats trained to discriminate 10 mg/kg chlordiazepoxide from saline (Krimmer, 1974b). The initial report that pentobarbital did not dependably elicit the drug response was in rats trained to discriminate the even higher chlordiazepoxide dose of 30 mg/kg from saline (Overton, 1966). Colpaert, Desmedt and Janssen (1976) found that pentobarbital elicited the drug response in rats trained to discriminate a low chlordiazepoxide dose (5 mg/kg) from its solvent at 30 minutes after oral administration. A partially differential effect of these drugs is suggested, however, by the approximately four-fold higher ED_{50} for pentobarbital (11.0 mg/kg) than for chlordiazepoxide (2.76 mg/kg).

The ED_{50} values for three drugs, shown in Table 1, may indicate some variations in the situation influencing the animal's sensitivity to the discriminative drug effects. The ED_{50} for chlordiazepoxide was highest (6.3 mg/kg) when animals were trained to discriminate alcohol from saline in a situation involving conflict between food-approach and shock-avoidance responses (Kubena and Barry, 1969b). This conflict situation might emphasize the differential effects of chlordiazepoxide. The ED_{50} for chlordiazepoxide was lowest (2.9 mg/kg) in animals trained to discriminate alcohol from saline at 20 rather than 5 minutes after injection (Krimmer, 1974b). Since chlordiazepoxide has slow-acting, long-lasting effects, it may resemble more closely the alcohol effect at the longer time after alcohol injection. The ED_{50} for pentobarbital was highest (12.3 mg/kg) in animals trained to discriminate alcohol from saline by turning in opposite directions in a T-maze for food (Bueno, Carlini, Finkelfarb and Suzuki, 1976). The response of running rather than pressing a lever might have enhanced the differential effects of the drugs.

According to the model (Fig. 3), bemegride increases both passivity and tension. Muscular tension is accompanied by passive inattention to environmental signals when this central nervous system stimulant is given in a dose sufficient to cause convulsions. The opposite effects of bemegride and pentobarbital, predicted from their positions in Figure 3, have been demonstrated by the use of bemegride to antagonize the drug response in animals trained to discriminate pentobarbital from saline. A shift from the drug to the saline response, when pentobarbital is combined with bemegride, has been reported in rats (Overton, 1966; Krimmer, 1974a; 1974b) and gerbils (Jarbe, Johansson and Henriksson, 1975; Johansson and Jarbe, 1975). Bemegride also antagonizes the drug response when combined with alcohol or pentobarbital in rats trained to discriminate alcohol from saline (Krimmer, 1974b) and when combined with chlordiazepoxide in rats trained to discriminate that drug from saline (Krimmer and Barry, unpublished).

Pentylenetetrazol (Metrazol) is also a central nervous system stimulant, causing convulsions at sufficient doses, but its position in Figure 3 indicates that it is less effective than bemegride as an antagonist of the discriminable effects of pentobarbital and especially alcohol. These differences between pentylenetetrazol and bemegride are consistent with experimental findings in rats (Krimmer, 1974a; 1974b) and in gerbils (Johansson and Jarbe, 1975). The model portrays pentylenetetrazol as causing an increase in passivity with no consistent effect on tension or sedation.

The position of amphetamine in Figure 3 is also consistent with experimental findings. Although this drug is classified as a central nervous system stimulant, it does not antagonize the discriminative effect of pentobarbital in rats (Krimmer, 1974a; 1974b) or in gerbils (Jarbe, Johansson and Henriksson, 1975). According to the model, amphetamine primarily increases arousal and thus shares one of the effects of pentobarbital. Amphetamine likewise did not antagonize the alcohol response in rats trained to discriminate alcohol (1000 mg/kg) from saline by pressing alternative levers for food (Krimmer, 1974a; 1974b). On the other hand, Schechter (1974) found that a high dose of amphetamine (4 mg/kg) partially antagonized the alcohol response in rats trained to discriminate a high alcohol dose (1500 mg/kg) from saline at 15 minutes after intraperitoneal injection. The differential response consisted of escaping shock by running in opposite directions from a central compartment into alternative compartments. The high doses might have enhanced the opposite effects of arousal caused by amphetamine and passivity caused by alcohol (Fig. 3). In the same study (Schechter, 1974), the alcohol response was not antagonized by propranolol or caffeine.

In an earlier study by Schechter (1973), with the same procedures, another treatment that antagonized the discriminative alcohol response gave evidence for the involvement of serotonin, a neurotransmitter, in the discriminative alcohol signal. A single oral dose of p-chlorophenylalanine (350 mg/kg), which depletes brain serotonin, caused the animals to choose the saline response for several weeks afterward, regardless of whether they were injected with alcohol or saline.

Chlorpromazine is represented in Figure 3 as increasing both sedation and passivity, in accordance with the general behavioral effects of this anti-psychotic agent. The discrimination between this drug and saline is difficult to train (Overton, 1966; Barry,

Steenberg, Manian and Buckley, 1974). The low degree of distinctiveness thereby indicated for chlorpromazine is attributable partly to the large amount of normal variation in the combined dimensions of sedation and passivity. High doses of chlorpromazine elicit the drug response to some degree in rats trained to discriminate alcohol from saline but not in rats trained to discriminate pentobarbital from saline (Krimmer, 1974b). This finding is consistent with the positions of these drugs in Figure 3.

In addition to the two dimensions portrayed in Figure 3, further attributes probably account for the discriminative effects of other categories of drugs, such as narcotic analgesics, antimuscarinics, hallucinogens, and cannabinoids. A review by Barry (1974) concluded that animals trained to discriminate a drug in one of these categories from the nondrug control condition generally choose the nondrug response in tests with drugs in other categories. Overton (1975) has reported evidence that the discriminative effects of two dissociative anesthetics, ketamine and phencyclidine, are partially differentiated from pentobarbital and from each other. On the other hand, similar discriminative effect have sometimes been reported for drugs in different categories. Jarbe and Henriksson (1974) found that rats trained to discriminate a very high dose of atropine (150 mg/kg) from saline, at 15 minutes after intraperitoneal injection, made the drug response in tests with pentobarbital (12.5 - 18.75 mg/kg). The discriminative response consisted of escaping from water by swimming in opposite directions in a T-maze.

VI. SUMMARY AND CONCLUSIONS

The effect of alcohol can be used as a conditional stimulus or discriminative signal for training rats to select differential responses on the basis of whether they have been administered alcohol or a control fluid. The dose has usually been 1000 - 1200 mg/kg, injected intraperitoneally between 5 and 20 minutes before the training sessions. Various incentives have been used, including food reward and shock escape. The performance learned by the animals has included alternative but equivalent responses, such as running in opposite directions or pressing alternative levers, and different types of responses, such as approach and avoidance.

Rats trained to discriminate alcohol from saline consistently select the drug response in tests with sufficiently high doses of other sedative-hypnotics, such as pentobarbital, and anti-anxiety agents, such as chlordiazepoxide. The discriminative alcohol effect is antagonized by bemegride, a central nervous stimulant. Other categories of drugs generally do not elicit or antagonize the alcohol response.

In rats trained to discriminate pentobarbital or chlordiazepoxide from saline, alcohol elicits the drug response only under some conditions. This evidence for partially different effects is supported by experiments in which rats were trained to discriminate alcohol from pentobarbital. Tests at other doses indicate that the discrimination was based on qualitatively different drug effects

and not merely on a quantitative difference in magnitude of the same
type of drug effect at the doses chosen by the experimenter.

The relationships among alcohol, pentobarbital, chlordiazepoxide,
and several other drugs, are portrayed by their positions on a model
of discriminative drug effects in terms of two dimensions, sedation-
tension and passivity-arousal. Alcohol increases sedation and to a
lesser degree increases passivity. Pentobarbital increases both
sedation and arousal. Chlordiazepoxide is intemediate between these
other two drugs.

The purpose of this model is to simplify the relationships among
the many types of drugs by defining the position of each drug on a
much smaller number of dimensions. A limited number of drugs can be
differentiated from each other on the basis of the two dimensions
defined. Additional dimensions are necessary to define the discriminative effects of other categories of drugs. It may be possible,
however, to differentiate among a large number of drug categories on
the basis of their positions on a small number of dimensions. This
is the model for discriminations among a wide variety of sensory
signals on the basis of their quantitative positions on a few
attributes. For example, an auditory discrimination among many
types of tones can be based on the three dimensions of frequency
(pitch), loudness, and duration.

Alcohol may be an appropriate prototype for the discriminative
effects of the sedative-hypnotic and anti-anxiety agents. Although
the discriminative effects of pentobarbital and chlordiazepoxide
appear to be more distinctive at doses with equivalent magnitudes of
effect on other types of behavior, the discriminative alcohol
response generalizes more consistently to these other drugs. The
discriminative effects of alcohol may be related to other attributes
of this drug, including its regular consumption by large numbers of
people in a wide variety of cultures.

VII. ACKNOWLEDGEMENTS

Preparation of this chapter was supported by U. S. Public
Health Service Research Scientist Development Award K2-MH-5921
(to H. B.), from the NIMH, by Post-Doctoral Research Fellowship
DA-2376 (to E. C. K.), from the NIDA, and by Research Grant
MH-13595 (to both authors), from the NIMH.

VIII. REFERENCES

Ando, K.: The discriminative control of operant behavior by
    intravenous administration of drugs in rats. Psychopharmacologia
    (Berl.) 45: 47-50, 1975.

Barry, H., III: Prolonged measurements of discrimination between
    alcohol and nondrug states. J. comp. physiol. Psychol.
    65: 349-352, 1968.

Barry, H., III: Classification of drugs according to their discriminable effects in rats. Fed. Proc. 33: 1814-1824, 1974.

Barry, H., III and Krimmer, E. C.: Pentobarbital effects perceived by rats as resembling several other depressants but not alcohol. Proc., 80th Ann. Convention, Amer. Psychol. Assoc. 7: 849-850, 1972.

Barry, H., III and Kubena, R. K.: Discriminative stimulus characteristics of alcohol, marihuana and atropine. In Drug Addiction, vol. 1, Experimental Pharmacology, ed. by J. M. Singh, L. H. Miller and H. Lal, pp. 3-16, Futura Publishing Co., Mt. Kisco, N. Y., 1972.

Barry, H., III, Koepfer, E. and Lutch, J.: Learning to discriminate between alcohol and nondrug condition. Psychol. Reports 16: 1072, 1965.

Barry, H., III, Steenberg, M. L., Manian, A. A. and Buckley, J. P.: Effects of chlorpromazine and three metabolites on behavioral responses in rats. Psychopharmacologia (Berl.) 34: 351-360, 1974.

Bueno, O. F. A., Carlini, E. A., Finkelfarb, E. and Suzuki, J. S.: Δ^9-Tetrahydrocannabinol, ethanol, and amphetamine as discriminative stimuli generalization tests with other drugs. Psychopharmacologia (Berl.) 46: 235-243, 1976.

Colpaert, F. C., Desmedt, L. K. C. and Janssen, P. A. J.: Discriminative stimulus properties of benzodiazepines, barbiturates and pharmacologically related drugs; relation to some intrinsic and anticonvulsant effects. Europ. J. Pharmacol. 37: 113-124, 1976.

Conger, J. J.: The effects of alcohol on conflict behavior in the albino rat. Quart. J. Stud. Alc. 12: 1-29, 1951.

Dollard, J. and Miller, N. E.: Personality and Psychotherapy. McGraw-Hill, New York, 1950.

Garcia, J., Hankins, W. G., Robinson, J. H. and Vogt, J. L.: Bait shyness: Tests of CS-US mediation. Physiol. and Behav. 8: 807-810, 1972.

Jarbe, T. U. C. and Henriksson, B. G.: Discriminative response control produced with hashish, tetrahydrocannabinols (Δ^8-THC and Δ^9-THC), and other drugs. Psychopharmacologia (Berl.) 40: 1-16, 1974.

Jarbe, T. U. C., Johansson, J. O. and Henriksson, B. G.: Δ^9-tetrahydrocannabinol and pentobarbital as discriminative cues in the Mongolian gerbil (Meriones unguiculatus). Physiol. Biochem. and Behav. 3: 403-410, 1975.

Johansson, J. O. and Jarbe, T. U. C.: Antagonism of pentobarbital induced discrimination in the gerbil. Psychopharmacologia (Berl.) 41: 225-228, 1975.

Kelleher, R. T.: Characteristics of behavior controlled by scheduled injections of drugs. Pharmacol. Rev. 27: 307-323, 1976.

Krimmer, E. C.: Selective antagonism of discriminable properties of pentobarbital by several stimulants. Fed. Proc. 33: 550, 1974a (Abstract).

Krimmer, E. C.: Drugs as Discriminative Stimuli. Ph.D. Dissertation, University of Pittsburgh, 1974b. Dissert. Abstr. Internat. 35: 4572-B (1974-75).

Krimmer, E. C. and Barry, H., III: Discriminability of pentobarbital and alcohol tested by two lever choice in shock escape. Pharmacologist 15: 236, 1973a (Abstract).

Krimmer, E. C. and Barry, H., III: Differential stimulus characteristics of alcohol and pentobarbital in rats. Proc. 81st Ann. Convention, Amer. Psychol. Assoc. 8: 1005-1006, 1973b.

Krimmer, E. C. and Barry, H., III: Discriminative pentobarbital stimulus in rats immediately after intravenous administration. Europ. J. Pharmacol. 38: 321-327, 1976.

Kubena, R. K. and Barry, H., III: Two procedures for training differential responses in alcohol and nondrug condition. J. Pham. Sci. 58: 99-101, 1969a.

Kubena, R. K. and Barry, H., III: Generalization by rats of alcohol and atropine stimulus characteristics to other drugs. Psychopharmacologia (Berl.) 15: 196-206, 1969b.

Overton, D. A.: Control of Learned Responses by Drug States. Ph.D. Dissertation, McGill University, 1962.

Overton, D. A.: State-dependent learning produced by depressant and atropine-like drugs. Psychopharmacologia (Berl.) 10: 6-31, 1966.

Overton, D. A.: State-dependent learning produced by alcohol and its relevance to alcoholism. In The Biology of Alcoholism, vol. 2, Physiology and Behavior, ed. by B. Kissin and H. Begleiter, pp. 193-217, Plenum Press, New York, 1972.

Overton, D. A.: A comparison of the discriminable CNS effects of ketamine, phencyclidine and pentobarbital. Arch. int. Pharmacodyn. 215: 180-189, 1975.

Pavlov. I. P.: Conditioned Reflexes. (Trans. by G. V. Anrep). Oxford Univer. Press, London, 1972.

Schechter, M. D.: Ethanol as a discriminative cue: Reduction following depletion of brain serotonin. Europ. J. Pharmacol. 24: 278-281, 1973.

Schechter, M. D.: Effect of propranol, d-amphetamine and caffeine on ethanol as a discriminative cue. Europ. J. Pharmacol. 29: 52-57, 1974.

Wallgren, H. and Barry, H., III: Actions of Alcohol, vol. 1, Biochemical, Physiological, and Psychological Aspects. Elsevier, Amsterdam, 1970.

Winter, J. C.: The stimulus properties of morphine and ethanol. Psychopharmacologia (Berl.) 44: 209-214, 1975.

DISCRIMINATIVE STIMULUS PROPERTIES OF BENZODIAZEPINES AND BARBITURATES

F.C. Colpaert

Dept. Pharmacology
Janssen Pharmaceutica Research Laboratories
B-2340 Beerse, Belgium

In the present chapter we will present and discuss some data on the discriminative stimulus properties of benzodiazepines and pharmacologically related drugs. The first set of data refers to stimulus generalization experiments with benzodiazepines, barbiturates and neuroleptics in rats trained to discriminate 5 mg/kg chlordiazepoxide from saline. The results obtained in that study (Colpaert et al., 1976b) are discussed in relation to a number of other pharmacologically relevant actions of the same drugs. A second set of data summarizes a large number of antagonism experiments the purpose of which was to identify somewhat more specifically the pharmacological action upon which the benzodiazepine cue is based. A major limitation of the results and conclusions presented here is, that they are derived from a single type of discrimination training (Colpaert et al., 1976a) with only one training dose (5 mg/kg) of one drug (chlordiazepoxide) administered orally 30 min before test.

I. DISCRIMINATIVE STIMULUS EQUIVALENCE

In rats trained as mentioned above, a large series of experiments was done to determine the possible discriminative stimulus equivalence of benzodiazepines (bromazepam, diazepam, flurazepam, lorazepam, nitrazepam, oxazepam), barbiturates (pentobarbital, phenobarbital, glutethimide) and neuroleptics (chlorpromazine, haloperidol) to 5 mg/kg chlordiazepoxide. The data are summarized in Fig. 1. It is shown that all benzodiazepines and barbiturates tested are generalized with chlordiazepoxide, whereas the neuroleptics chlorpromazine and haloperidol are not. This result indicates that the cuing properties of benzodiazepines and barbiturates are pharmacologically specific.

As a first step to identify the pharmacological action underlying the benzodiazepine cue, we have established the statistical relations of the cuing properties of these drugs to some of their intrinsic and anticonvulsant effects (Colpaert et al., 1976b). These effects include: induction of ataxia (ATA) and loss of the righting reflex (LRR), and antagonism to pentylenetetrazol-induced tonic hind paw extension (THP), tonic forepaw extension (TFP), generalized clonic seizures (CLO) and tremors (TRE). It follows (Table 1) that the

Table 1. Intercorrelation between discriminative stimulus properties (CUE), intrinsic behavioral effects (ATA, LRR) and anticonvulsant (CLO, TFP, THP, TRE) activity of benzodiazepines and barbiturates (*: $p < .01$; **: $p < .001$)

	CLO	ATA	TFP	THP	TRE	LRR
CUE	.95 **	.90 **	.90 **	.73 *	.33	.03
CLO		.98 **	.98 **	.79 *	.38	.08
ATA			.98 **	.85 **	.41	.09
TFP				.84 **	.41	.07
THP					.52	.26
TRE						.79 *

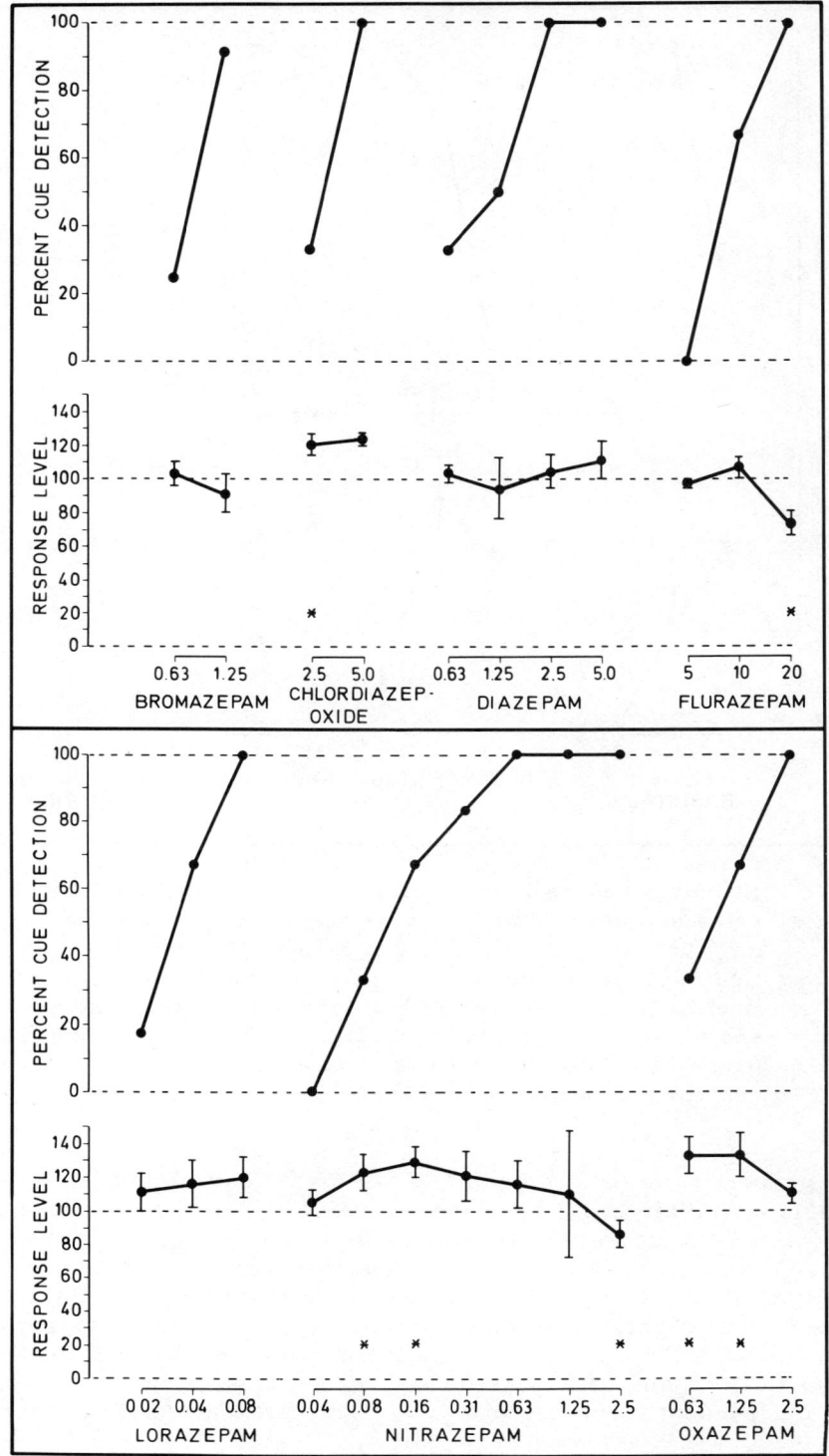

Fig. 1

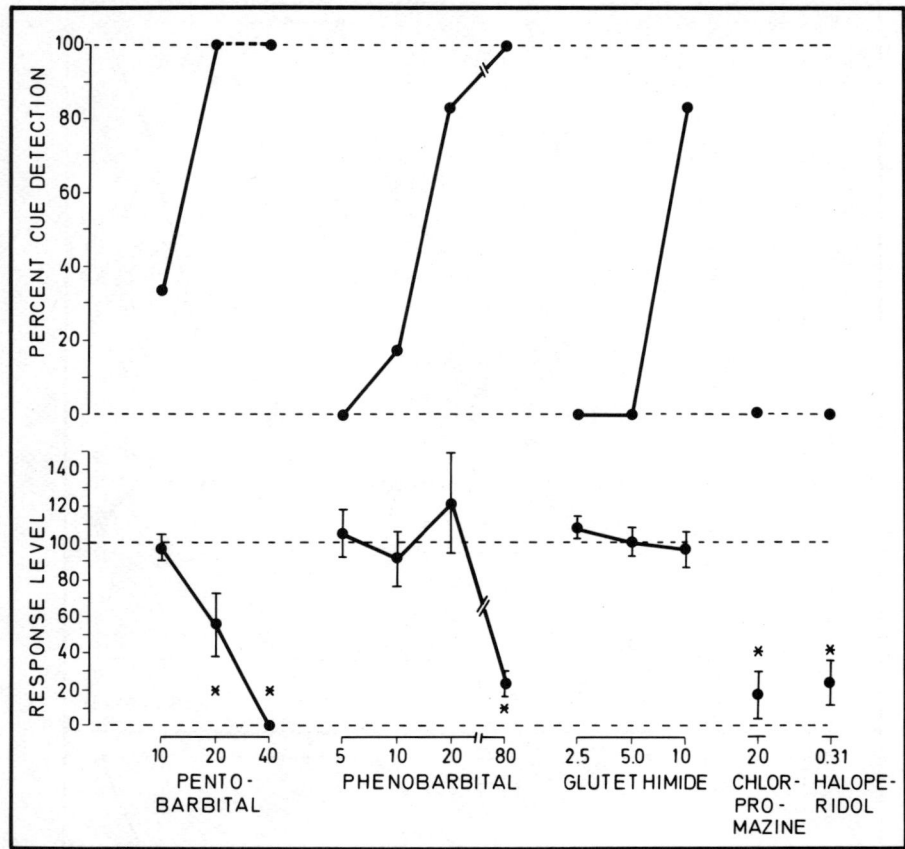

Fig. 1. Stimulus generalization with benzodiazepines, barbitu-
(cont'd) rates and neuroleptics in rats trained to discriminate 5
mg/kg chlordiazepoxide from saline. Percent cue detection represents the percentage of animals which generalize the test treatment with chlordiazepoxide. The response level refers to the total amount of responding (bar-
pressing for food), expressed as a percentage of saline-
control performance (*: $p < .05$).

cuing properties of benzodiazepines are highly correlated ($r_s = .90$;
$p < .001$) with their capacity to induce ataxia, as well as with their
antagonistic effects to pentylenetetrazol-induced clonic seizures
($r_s = .95$; $p < .001$). These two correlations are represented gra-
phically in Figs 2 and 3. The picture which emerges from Table 1
is that CUE is highly correlated with a cluster of 3 other variables
(CLO, ATA, TFP) which show significant correlations (.79 to .85)
with THP; TRE and LRR constitute a second cluster which is essentially independent from the first one. Spectral Map Analysis on the

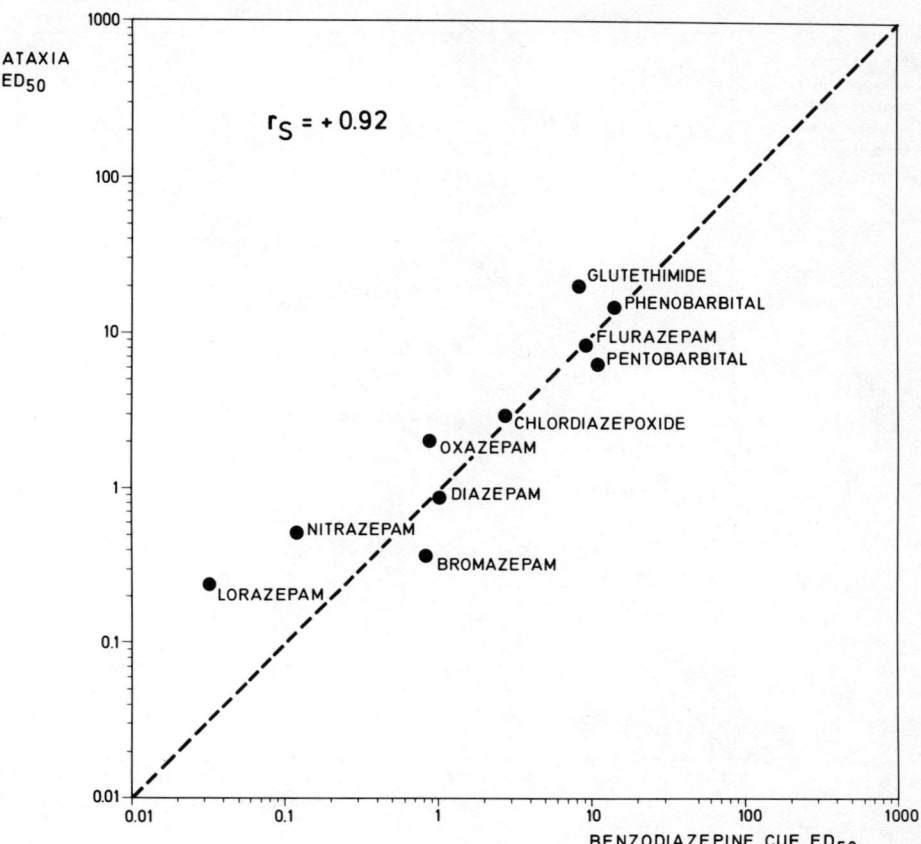

Fig. 2. Relation between cuing properties and ataxia-inducing effects

basis of the ED_{50} values of the 7 benzodiazepines and 3 barbiturates in the tests for intrinsic (ATA, LRR) and anticonvulsant (CLO, TFP, THP, TRE) activity confirms (Fig. 4) that these parameters are organized along 3 poles (CLO-ATA-TFP; TRE-LRR; THP). The total power of this representation is 96 %, thus indicating that the analysis accounts for virtually all the variability of the data. Addition of the cuing effects to the data pool submitted to the Spectral Map Analysis reveals (Fig. 5) that these cuing effects define a novel pole at the expense of the THP parameter. As much as 92 % of the variability is accounted for by this analysis. This result indicates that the cuing properties of benzodiazepines and barbiturates constitute a relevant dimension in the pharmacological activity profile of these drugs.

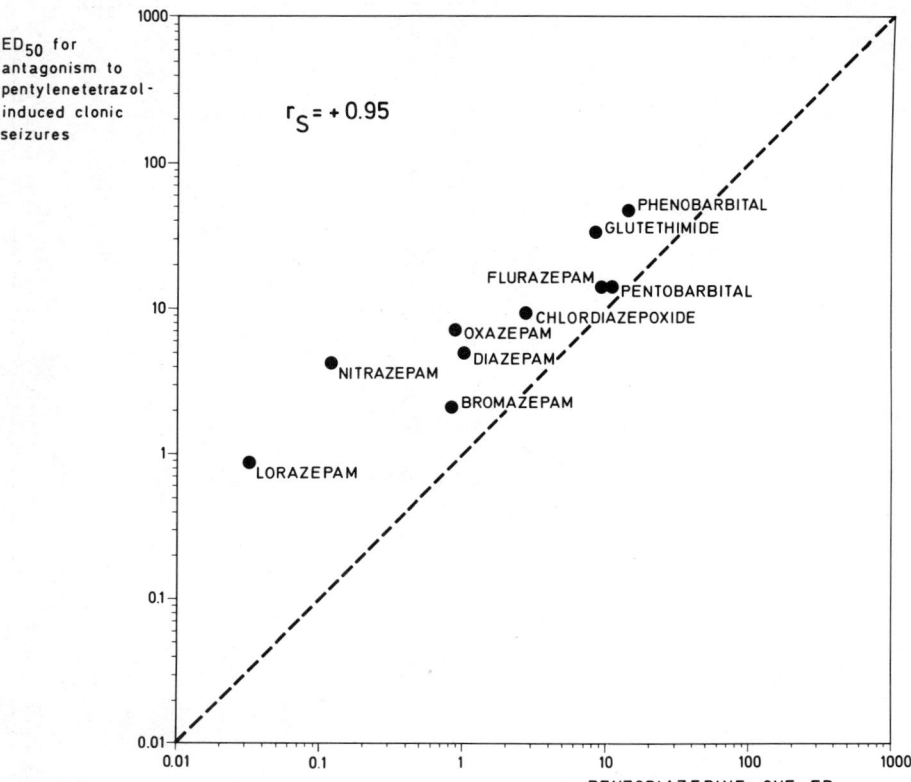

Fig. 3. Relation between cuing properties and antagonism of pentylenetetrazol-induced clonic seizures

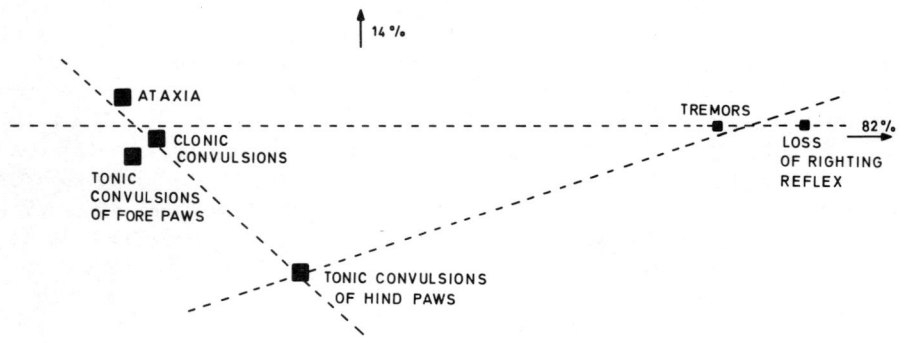

Fig. 4. Spectral Map Analysis of intrinsic (ATA, LRR) and anticonvulsant (CLO, TFP, THP, TRE) activity of 7 benzodiazepines and 3 barbiturates.

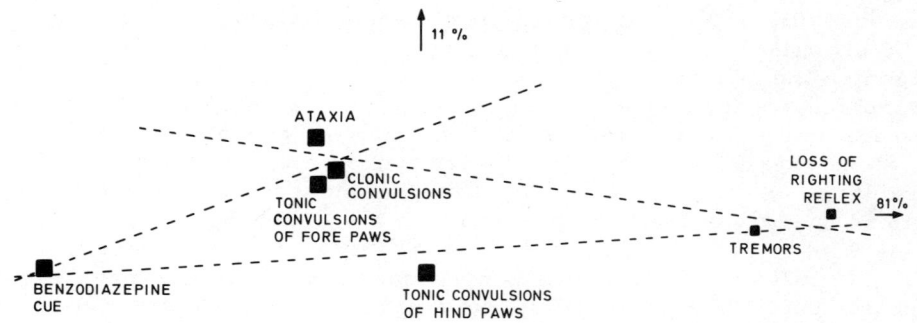

Fig. 5. Spectral Map Analysis of cuing (CUE), intrinsic (ATA, LRR) and anticonvulsant (CLO, TFP, THP, TRE) activity of 7 benzodiazepines and 3 barbiturates

II. ANTAGONISM OF THE BENZODIAZEPINE CUE

The biochemical, pharmacological and behavioral actions of benzodiazepines and barbiturates are numerous and heterogenous, and to find out which action(s) is responsible for the cuing properties of these drugs is a difficult task. In pharmacology, a commonly practiced strategy to tackle this type of problems consists of searching an effective antagonist for the action being studied, and this approach has led us to examine the possible effects of a large series of potential antagonists, on the benzodiazepine cue. Rats were trained to discriminate 5 mg/kg chlordiazepoxide (p.o., t-30') from saline as described previously (Colpaert et al., 1976a); in addition to this discriminandum, the animals were always given a subcutaneous (t-30') saline injection. On test sessions, the latter saline injection was substituted for by test treatment.

Three types of compounds were studied for possible antagonism (see Tables 2 to 4), and the doses applied were selected on the basis of discriminability and toxicity. That is, only drugs which, in preliminary experiments, had been found to possess intrinsic discriminative stimulus properties, were considered for test. The doses used were those which had been found to be subtoxic at either the behavioral or the physiological level.

The results obtained with CNS stimulant and/or psychotomimetic drugs are summarized in Table 2. Apomorphine (0.16 mg/kg) and dl-amphetamine (0.63 mg/kg) antagonized benzodiazepine cue detection in one out of 6 animals; the higher apomorphine dose (0.63 mg/kg) suppressed responding completely, whereas 2.5 mg/kg amphetamine failed to produce any antagonism. No antagonism was observed after caffeine (40 and 160 mg/kg), cocaine (5 and 20 mg/kg)

or mescaline (10 and 40 mg/kg) and it seems fair to conclude that CNS stimulant and/or psychotomimetic drugs do not effectively antagonize the benzodiazepine cue. However, the findings with apomorphine are inconclusive, and further work is required to clarify its possible effects on the cuing properties of benzodiazepines.
A second series of drugs tested were typical analeptic compounds (Table 3). Bemegride (0.63 to 10 mg/kg) antagonized the benzodiazepine cue in a dose-related way (ED_{50} = 4.05 mg/kg; 95 % C.L.: 1.39-11.8); these are fairly low doses of this drug, and no statistically significant effects on total response output were obtained (response level 106.8 to 86.3 %). No antagonism whatsoever was observed following isoniazid (40 and 160 mg/kg), pentylenetetrazol (10 and 40 mg/kg), picrotoxin (0.16 and 0.63 mg/kg), strychnine (0.16 and 0.63 mg/kg) or tryptamine (10 and 40 mg/kg).
The third series of drugs tested consisted of cholinergic agents (Table 4). Carbachol (0.08 and 0.31 mg/kg), neostigmine (0.04 and 0.16 mg/kg) and physostigmine (0.04 and 0.16 mg/kg) showed no antagonism. Tremorine (5 and 20 mg/kg) antagonized benzodiazepine cue detection in one out of six animals; due to acute lethal effects, higher doses of this drug could not be tested. A dose-related (ED_{50} = 0.32 mg/kg; 95 % C.L.: 0.12-0.83) antagonism of the benzodiazepine cue was produced by nicotine (0.04 to 0.63 mg/kg); at its highest dose, the percentage of total response output on the selected lever was significantly deteriorated. The latter does not seem to be due to unspecific behavioral toxicity, as no effects on total amount of responding were observed.

From the present experiments it can be concluded that, out of all CNS stimulant, psychotomimetic, analeptic and cholinergic compounds tested, only bemegride and nicotine are effective antagonists of the benzodiazepine cue. The deleterious effect of nicotine on response accuracy suggests that its antagonistic action is somewhat less specific than that of bemegride.

III. GENERAL DISCUSSION

That benzodiazepines and barbiturates possess discriminative stimulus properties is well established now. Stimulus generalization experiments (Fig. 1) in rats trained to discriminate 5 mg/kg chlordiazepoxide from saline reveal that these drugs (7 benzodiazepines and 3 barbiturates tested) produce a discriminative stimulus complex, or cue, which is similar to that of chlordiazepoxide. It is also apparent that there is no relation between the cuing and the rate-altering effects of these drugs; increase, decrease, or no change of total response output may accompany stimulus generalization. Under these conditions, stimulus generalization appears to be dose-dependent; supramaximal doses (e.g. 5 mg/kg diazepam, 1.25 and 2.5 mg/kg nitrazepam, 80 mg/kg phenobarbital) elicit 100 % genera-

Table 2. Effects of CNS stimulant and/or psychotomimetic drugs on the benzodiazepine cue. Symbols: n_t = number of rats tested; n-SL/n_r = number of rats selecting the saline lever out of the number of rats which showed any responding at all. FRF reflects accuracy of lever selection. The asterisk denotes $p < .05$ for the response level data

Compound	Dose (mg/kg)	n_t	n-SL/n_r	FRF		% of TR on selected lever		Response level	
dl-amphetamine	0.63	6	1/6	10	(10-15)	100	(99.5-100)	128.1*	(±6.8)
dl-amphetamine	2.5	6	0/6	10	(10-12)	99.8	(98.7-100)	79.1	(±13.4)
apomorphine	0.16	6	1/6	10	(10-13)	98.8	(61.8-100)	55.8*	(±12.5)
apomorphine	0.63	6	0/0	—		—		0.2*	(±0.1)
caffeine	40	6	0/6	10	(10-10)	99.8	(77.5-100)	87.0	(±7.3)
caffeine	160	6	0/3	10	(10-11)	99.7	(80.8-100)	34.8*	(±16.2)
cocaine	5	6	0/6	10	(10-10)	99.9	(99.6-100)	143.0*	(±9.0)
cocaine	20	6	0/6	10	(10-10)	100	(99.4-100)	134.0*	(±6.3)
mescaline	10	6	0/6	10	(10-11)	99.9	(97.8-100)	122.3*	(±8.2)
mescaline	40	5	0/5	10	(10-10)	100	(100-100)	95.9	(±5.1)

Table 3. Effects of typical analeptic drugs on the benzodiazepine cue

Compound	Dose (mg/kg)	n_t	n-SL n_r	FRF		% of TR on selected lever		Response level	
bemegride	0.63	6	0/6	10	(10-11)	100	(99.7-100)	106.8	(±5.7)
bemegride	2.5	6	2/6	10	(10-11)	100	(99.5-100)	102.4	(±10.1)
bemegride	10	6	5/6	10	(10-12)	99.9	(98.9-100)	86.3	(±8.5)
isoniazid	40	5	0/5	10	(10-10)	100	(100-100)	116.0	(±10.2)
isoniazid	160	5	0/5	10	(10-10)	100	(99.9-100)	109.0	(±4.8)
pentylenetetrazol	10	6	0/6	10	(10-10)	100	(99.5-100)	122.1	(±14.1)
pentylenetetrazol	40	6	0/6	10	(10-10)	100	(100-100)	51.7*	(±7.6)
picrotoxin	0.16	4	0/4	10	(10-10)	100	(100-100)	107.8	(±7.8)
picrotoxin	0.63	5	0/5	10	(10-10)	100	(100-100)	110.1	(±3.9)
strychnine	0.16	6	0/6	10	(10-10)	100	(99.9-100)	110.2	(±10.0)
strychnine	0.63	6	0/6	10	(10-10)	100	(100-100)	117.7*	(±5.9)
tryptamine	10	6	0/6	10	(10-10)	100	(100-100)	106.5	(±5.4)
tryptamine	40	5	0/5	10	(10-11)	100	(99.9-100)	97.8	(±19.1)

Table 4. Effects of cholinergic agents on the benzodiazepine cue

Compound	Dose (mg/kg)	n_t	n-SL $\frac{n_r}{}$	FRF		% of TR on selected lever		Response level	
carbachol	0.08	5	0/5	10	(10-10)	100	(99.9-100)	95.1	(±4.9)
carbachol	0.31	5	0/5	10	(10-10)	100	(100-100)	79.3	(±8.8)
neostigmine	0.04	4	0/4	10	(10-10)	100	(100-100)	119.0	(±13.4)
neostigmine	0.16	5	0/5	10	(10-15)	99.9	(99.2-100)	89.0	(±9.6)
nicotine	0.04	5	0/5	10	(10-10)	100	(100-100)	113.0	(±18.0)
nicotine	0.16	6	1/6	10	(10-13)	100	(99.5-100)	106.4	(±5.5)
nicotine	0.63	6	5/6	10	(10-11)	97.3*	(90.2-99.9)	123.2	(±12.0)
physostigmine	0.04	5	0/5	10	(10-10)	100	(99.9-100)	107.4	(±6.1)
physostigmine	0.16	4	0/4	10	(10-10)	100	(71.3-100)	88.1	(±5.5)
tremorine	5	6	1/6	10	(10-10)	100	(92.0-100)	80.0	(±16.2)
tremorine	20	6	1/6	10	(10-11)	99.2	(86.2-100)	35.7*	(±12.8)

lization, thus suggesting that the qualitative properties of the cuing effects of these drugs at relatively high doses do not significantly, if at all, differ from those associated with lower doses.

All compounds which were found to be generalized with the benzodiazepine cue, also produce ataxia, and there is a close correlation between the two phenomena (Fig. 2). However, ataxia itself does not constitute the benzodiazepine cue, as some of these compounds produce the cue at doses far below those required to produce ataxia (Colpaert et al., 1976b). The fact that the cuing properties of benzodiazepines are closely correlated with some of their major intrinsic effects (i.e. ataxia), strongly favors the position that these properties constitute a pharmacologically specific and relevant drug action. This position is corroborated by further comparative data (Table 1) showing that the cuing properties of the benzodiazepines and barbiturates are also correlated with part of the anticonvulsant activity of these drugs. Antagonism of pentylenetetrazol-induced generalized clonic seizures is a major characteristic of the pharmacological activity profile of these drugs (Fig. 4), and this parameter shows an extremely high correlation ($r_s = .95$; $p < .001$) with cuing effects (Fig. 3).

Although these correlations substantiate the pharmacological specificity of the benzodiazepine cue, they do not indicate that these cuing properties would constitute a redundant measurement of benzodiazepine and barbiturate drug activity. Spectral Map Analysis is a statistical method which aims to identify the major dimensions along which the variability which occurs within a given data pool, can be defined. This analysis shows (Fig. 5) that the measurement of the cuing properties of benzodiazepines and barbiturates adds significantly new information to the known activity profile of these compounds. The possible clinical relevance of this finding remains to be determined.

With respect to the antagonism experiments (Tables 2 to 4), the following consideration seems in place; a drug may conceivably antagonize the cuing properties of another compound in one of two ways. One way is by affecting the physiological process(es) underlying the agonist drugs' cuing effects. Another is by "overriding" these effects; that is, the presumed antagonist may possess intrinsic cuing effects of such distinctiveness that those of the compound being studied are no longer detectable for the animal. It is somewhat surprising to find out, therefore, that only two out of the 16 compounds tested, antagonized the benzodiazepine cue, despite the fact that all these 16 compounds had been found to exert intrinsic cuing effects. This finding seems to argue against the second alternative for cue antagonism, although the exact basis for that by bemegride and nicotine has not yet been clarified. At present, no comparative data on the absolute discriminability of bemegride, nicotine and chlordiazepoxide or on that of appropriate combinations of these drugs are available. Bemegride antagonism has formerly been observed by Overton (1966) on rats trained on 10 mg/kg pentobarbital, the ED_{50} value amounting to 20-25 mg/kg. Jarbe et al. (1975) likewise found that, in gerbils, 20 to 40 mg/kg bemegride antagonizes 20 mg/kg

pentobarbital. Of more interest to the present issue is the fact that
20 mg/kg bemegride attenuates the discriminability of 8 mg/kg diazepam (Johansson and Järbe, 1975a) as well as that of 15 mg/kg
pentobarbital (Johansson and Järbe, 1975b). This strongly suggests
that antagonism between benzodiazepines and barbiturates on the one
hand, and bemegride on the other, is based upon actions which conflict at the physiological rather than at the "distinctiveness" level.
The antagonism may be mutual, as bemegride does produce a cue
(unpublished results) but, again, appropriate comparative data are
required to substantiate this point.
In view of these data it seems reasonable to assume that the bemegride antagonism to the cuing properties of benzodiazepines and
barbiturates is pharmacologically specific. The nature of the nicotine antagonism remains to be elucidated.

The finding that the CNS stimulants dl-amphetamine, caffeine
and cocaine fail to antagonize the cuing properties of benzodiazepines,
supports the hypothesis (Colpaert et al., 1976b) that these properties
are not subserved by the general sedative or depressant action of
these drugs. Also, in our procedure, 40 mg/kg cocaine (s.c.) has
considerably higher discriminability than 5 mg/kg (p.o.) chlordiazepoxide, and this particular case strongly argues against a possible
"overriding" effect as a basis to explain cue antagonism.
The finding that the GABA biosynthesis inhibitor isoniazid, the GABA
blocker picrotoxin, the glycine blocker strychnine and the serotonergic agonist tryptamine, do not antagonize the benzodiazepine cue,
further narrows the potential action field involved in this cue. The
lack of antagonism with pentylenetetrazol is consistent with earlier
findings (Johansson and Järbe, 1975b) indicating that this drug is a
relatively ineffective antagonist of pentobarbital in gerbils as well.
Nevertheless, the differential effects of bemegride and pentylenetetrazol on the benzodiazepine cue remain puzzling in view of the fact
that these two drugs are generally considered to exert very similar
pharmacological effects (Hahn, 1960). The fact that nicotine, but not
the 4 other cholinergic agents tested, antagonizes the benzodiazepine
cue, points to a specific nicotinic-cholinergic involvement in this cue.
This is consistent with the presumed (Aceto, 1975) relevance of the
antinicotinic effects of benzodiazepines, barbiturates and related
compounds to their clinical action. Obviously, more data are needed
to determine the precise role of the antinicotinic effects of these
drugs in their cuing properties.

IV. CONCLUSION

The discriminative stimulus properties of benzodiazepines
and barbiturates constitute an interesting and pharmacologically
specific phenomenon. The data discussed here may contribute to an
identification of the physiological action(s) underlying the benzodiaze-

pine cue, and some findings (such as the antagonism by bemegride and nicotine) seem to provide valuable leads for further experimental analysis. The relevance of the benzodiazepine cue to the clinical effects of these and pharmacologically related drugs, remains to be determined.

V. REFERENCES

ACETO, M.D.: The antinicotinic effects of drugs with clinically useful sedative-antianxiety properties. Pharmacology 13: 458-464, 1975.

COLPAERT, F.C., NIEMEGEERS, C.J.E. AND JANSSEN, P.A.J.: Theoretical and methodological considerations on drug discrimination learning. Psychopharmacologia 46: 169-177, 1976a.

COLPAERT, F.C., DESMEDT, L.K.C. AND JANSSEN, P.A.J.: Discriminative stimulus properties of benzodiazepines, barbiturates and pharmacologically related drugs; relation to some intrinsic and anticonvulsant effects. Eur. J. Pharmacol. 37: 113-123, 1976b.

HAHN, F.: Analeptics. Pharmacol. Rev. 12: 447-530, 1960.

JÄRBE, T.U.C., JOHANSSON, J.O. AND HENRIKSSON, B.G.: Δ 9-tetrahydrocannabinol and pentobarbital as discriminative cues in the mongolian gerbil (Meriones unguiculatus). Pharmacol. Biochem. Behav. 3: 403-410, 1975.

JOHANSSON, J.O. AND JÄRBE, T.U.C.: Diazepam as a discriminative cue: its antagonism by bemegride. Eur. J. Pharmacol. 30: 372-375, 1975a.

JOHANSSON, J.O. AND JÄRBE, T.U.C.: Antagonism of pentobarbital induced discrimination in the gerbil. Psychopharmacologia 41: 225-228, 1975b.

OVERTON, D.A.: State-dependent learning produced by depressant and atropine-like drugs. Psychopharmacologia 10: 6-31, 1966.

CHARACTERIZATION OF DISCRIMINATIVE RESPONSE CONTROL BY PSYCHOMOTOR STIMULANTS

Peter B. Silverman and Beng T. Ho

Texas Research Institute of Mental Sciences
and
The University of Texas Health Science Center at Houston,
Houston, Texas   77030

I. INTRODUCTION

Among the drugs which effectively control discriminative responding are the psychomotor stimulants. Despite differences in methodology utilized in different laboratories, the results available to date are quite consistent. Amphetamine, the prototype of this class of drugs, has been most extensively studied. For this reason, our discussion will center on amphetamine, other stimulants being mentioned where data are available.

II. METHODOLOGY

Since results are generally similar without regard to the method used to obtain them, methods will be discussed only briefly. Similar findings with diverse methodology demonstrate the robust nature of the discriminative response-control by stimulant drugs.

Basically, an animal is injected with drug solution or solvent at a fixed period of time before being placed in a choice situation. In sessions following drug administration one of the two responses is reinforced while in sessions following solvent administration the other response is reinforced. The animal must learn to discriminate the presence of drug from its absence in order to gain reinforcement. In addition to the drug versus solvent discrimination, animals can be trained to discriminate between two drugs or two doses of the same drug. Methodological differences lie in the choice situation provided. In the first method a differential rate ("go, no-go") procedure is utilized. A one-lever operant chamber is the apparatus. Under one drug condition (e.g., presence or absence) responding is positively reinforced according to a standard operant schedule. In the opposite condition responding is not reinforced or is punished usually according to the same schedule. Since most centrally active drugs have effects on operant response rate, half of the subjects must be trained with the drug condition associated with positive reinforcement and the remaining half of the subjects trained with the drug associated with no reinforcement (or punishment). Acquisition of the discrimination is assessed in the training sessions which begin with a brief extinction period during which responses have no consequences. To test a novel condition, the short extinction period is not followed by the remaining training session.

In a second method, animals escape from electric footshock in a T-maze or similar apparatus. Termination of the shock is dependent on entry into the arm of the maze paired with the imposed drug condition. A number of trials are given in daily sessions and acquisition of the discrimination is assessed by the arm entered by the subject on the first trial of each session. Testing of novel conditions consists of a single trial in which entry into either arm of the maze terminates the shock.

In the third method, the experimental space is a two-lever operant chamber. Responding on one lever is reinforced following drug administration, while responding on the other is reinforced following solvent administration. Acquisition of discriminated responding is measured by the proportion of responses on the lever appropriate for the drug condition in brief extinction periods at the beginning of training sessions. Tests of novel conditions consist of extinction periods alone.

Variants of these three procedures exist and a variety of reinforcers and schedules have been used in the two operant procedures. Most of the papers reviewed here used either a T-maze or two-lever operant chamber method.

III. GENERAL PROPERTIES OF THE PSYCHOMOTOR STIMULANT CUE

Locus of cue

Only a few findings have direct bearing on the locus of the cue produced by stimulants. Schechter and Rosecrans (1972) trained animals to discriminate 4 mg/kg (+)-amphetamine from saline. Responding similar to the training dose of amphetamine was produced by 8 mg/kg (-)-amphetamine while some deficit in amphetamine appropriate responding followed administration of 4 mg/kg (-)-amphetamine. Jones *et al* (1974) found that in animals trained with 0.8 mg/kg (+)-amphetamine, 0.8 mg/kg of (-)-amphetamine produced essentially random responding while 1.6 mg/kg of the (-)-isomer generalized to the drug training condition. Since the isomers of amphetamine are equipotent in the periphery (Innes and Nickerson, 1975), these findings suggest a CNS locus for the mediation of the amphetamine cue. Jones *et al* (1974) further found that *para*-hydroxyamphetamine (1.01 mg/kg) was incapable of serving as a discriminative stimulus and at 1.01 and 2.02 mg/kg did not produce amphetamine appropriate responding in animals trained on 0.8 mg/kg (+)- or (-)-amphetamine. This further suggests a CNS locus since *para*-hydroxyamphetamine has peripheral activity similar to amphetamine but it possesses little (if any) central action due to its limited ability to cross the blood-brain barrier. Richards *et al* (1973) found that an intraventricularly administered dose of as little as 100 μg (+)-amphetamine generalized to a training dose of 1.5 mg/kg (i.p.). A CNS locus of the amphetamine cue is again implied. There seem to be no reports of more specific localization within the CNS.

Preliminary studies from our lab indicate CNS mediation of the discriminative stimulus resulting from cocaine administration. Ten and 20 mg/kg of quarternary cocaine, which does not cross the blood-brain barrier, produced saline responding in animals trained to discriminate 10 mg/kg cocaine from saline (Ho and McKenna, 1976).

Time Course

Degree of amphetamine control of operant responding as a function of the injection to test interval has been examined in three studies with similar results (Huang and Ho, 1974; Kuhn *et al*, 1974; Jones *et al*, 1976). All show that when tested with the same dose used in training, responding is appropriate for the drug condition for about one hour, reaching chance (50%) levels between 90 minutes and two hours, and is thereafter appropriate for saline. Jones *et al*, (1976) showed that a dose higher than the training dose results in amphetamine appropriate responding at longer intervals. When tested with the training dose immediately after injection for a ten minute period, Jones *et al*, (1976) found from 45 to 60% of total responses on the drug lever. Kuhn *et al* (1974) reported that their subjects responded on the drug appropriate lever immediately after drug injection.

Animals trained to discriminate 3.0 mg/kg methylphenidate from saline made less than 20% drug appropriate responses when tested immediately after injection for three minutes. When tested five minutes after injection for three minutes, about 80% of responses were on the drug lever. Like amphetamine, most responses were on the drug lever when tested at one hour post-injection and the saline lever when tested at two hours post-injection (Silverman and Ho, in preparation).

The rapid onset of stimulant control after i.p. injection is an interesting finding. Since one would expect uneven distribution of the drug in the brain at these short intervals, examination of drug distribution may provide information on brain loci involved in drug discrimination performance.

Dose response curves

Dose response curves for amphetamine trained animals have been generated in a number of studies (Huang and Ho, 1974c; Kuhn *et al*, 1974; Schechter and Cook, 1975; Tilson *et al*, 1975; Waters *et al*, 1972). All demonstrate that response control is not an all-or-none phenomenon but a graded effect. Curves produced by plotting percent amphetamine appropriate responding versus percent of training dose tested show good agreement between studies regardless of training procedure or training dose used. Barry (1974) suggests use of an ED_{50} to describe drug potency. The ED_{50} for amphetamine is clearly dependent on the dose used in original training.

Dose response curves for cocaine and methylphenidate have been generated in our lab. These curves are much steeper than our amphetamine curve but are not much different from the amphetamine dose response relationship obtained by other investigators (Figure 1).

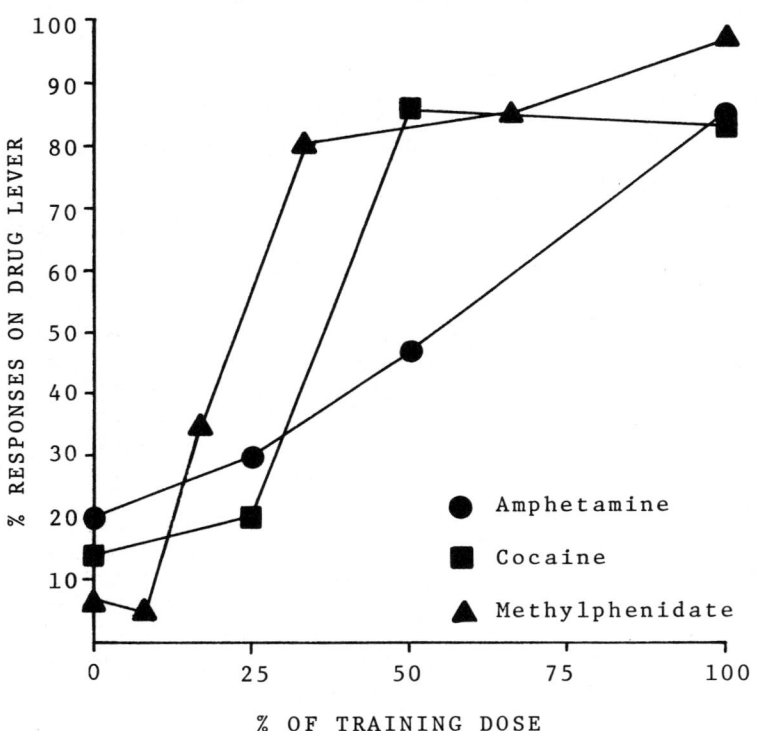

Figure 1. Dose response curves for three stimulants in two-lever operant paradigm. Training doses: amphetamine 0.8 mg/kg, cocaine 10 mg/kg, methylphenidate 3 mg/kg. Amphetamine and cocaine curves were generated in 10-minute extinction tests, DRL 15-sec schedule; methylphenidate 3-minute test, FR20 schedule.

Specificity of stimulant response control

A good deal of data has been generated which clearly demonstrates that animals trained to discriminate a stimulant injection from a saline injection are not merely responding along a "drugged-not-drugged" continuum. The specificity of discriminative control exerted by stimulants is demonstrated in several ways. First, animals trained to discriminate drugs other than stimulants from saline make predominantly saline-appropriate responses when tested with stimulants, i.e., stimulants do not produce generalization to other agents. A number of such agents are shown in Table 1. Secondly, the converse also holds true; when a stimulant is used as the training drug, agents other than stimulants do not produce generalization. This is shown in Table 2.

In contrast to findings with agents from other drug classes, animals trained with one psychomotor stimulant show response generalization when tested with other stimulants. These findings are summarized in Table 3.

Table 1. Nongeneralization of psychomotor stimulants to drug responding

Training Drug [mg/kg]	Test Drug [mg/kg]	References
Ethanol [1,200]	(+)-Amphetamine [1, 2]	13
Pentobarbital [20]	(+)-Amphetamine [2.5-10]	33
LSD [0.048]	(+)-Amphetamine [2, 4]	20
Mescaline [10]	(+)-Amphetamine [1] Cocaine [30]	30
Nicotine [0.2]	(+)-Amphetamine [0.4]	15
Nicotine [0.4]	(+)-Amphetamine [2, 4]	21
THC [4]	Methamphetamine [1.0] Cocaine [10, 20]	2

Table 2. Drugs which do not generalize to psychomotor stimulants

Training Drug [mg/kg]	Test Drug [mg/kg]	References
(+)-Amphetamine [1]	Atropine [10]	3
(+)-Amphetamine [4]	Nicotine [0.4] Fenfluramine [4-8] Mescaline [7.4-29.7] LSD [0.048]	22
(+)-Amphetamine [0.8]	p-Hydroxyamphetamine [1.01]	12
(−)-Amphetamine [0.8]	p-Hydroxyamphetamine [1.01, 2.02]	12
(+)-Amphetamine [0.8]	Iproniazid [100] β-Phenylethylamine [1]	7
(+)-Amphetamine [0.8]	3-Methoxyamphetamine [2, 4] 2,5-Dimethoxyamphetamine [1-4] 4-Methylamphetamine [1, 2] 4-Hydroxyamphetamine [1, 2] 2,5-Dimethoxy-4-methylamphetamine (STP) [0.25-1] 2,5-Dimethoxy-4-ethylamphetamine (DOET) [0.25-0.5] Mescaline [12.5, 25] Tyramine [1, 4] Oxotremorine [0.1, 0.25]	9
(+)-Amphetamine [1]	LSD [0.04, 0.08] Psilocybin [0.5, 1] Mescaline [5, 10] THC [0.5, 1] Caffeine [6, 20]	14
(+)-Amphetamine [0.8]	Nikethamide [25-75] Picrotoxin [1, 2] Strychnine [0.5, 1]	8
(+)-Amphetamine [0.8]	Amantadine [25, 50]	4

Table 3. Drugs which generalize to psychomotor stimulants

Training Drug [mg/kg]	Test Drug [mg/kg]	References
(±)-Amphetamine [1]	(+)-Amphetamine [1] Methylphenidate [4.5]	3
(+)-Amphetamine [4]	(−)-Amphetamine [8]	22
(−)-Amphetamine [0.8]	(+)-Amphetamine [0.8]	12
(+)-Amphetamine [0.8]	(−)-Amphetamine [1.6, 2.4]	12
(+)-Amphetamine [0.8]	Iproniazid [100] + β-Phenylethylamine [1]	7
(+)-Amphetamine [0.8]	(−)-Amphetamine [1.6] Methamphetamine [0.8, 1.6] 4-Methoxyamphetamine [2] Ephedrine [8.0] Norephedrine [8.0] Methylphenidate [2.5] Cocaine [7.5]	9
(+)-Amphetamine	Methamphetamine [1]	14
(+)-Amphetamine [3.0]	Apomorphine [1.25-5]	19
(+)-Amphetamine [0.8]	Ro 4-4602 [50] + L-DOPA [100] Ro 4-4602 [50] + amantadine [25, 50] + L-DOPA [100]	4
(+)-Amphetamine [1]	(−)-2,5-Dimethoxy-4-methylamphetamine (STP) [0.5, 0.75]	27
Cocaine [10]	(+)-Amphetamine [0.8] Methylphenidate [2.5] Propranolol [15]	5
Methylphenidate [3]	(+)-Amphetamine [0.5, 1] Cocaine [7.5]	25

Among the more ambiguous results are those obtained with 2,5-dimethoxy-4-methylamphetamine (DOM, STP). Huang (1972) was unable to train animals in a two-lever discrimination using doses of 0.5 or 0.8 mg/kg (±)-DOM versus saline. Huang and Ho (1974c) found that animals trained on 0.8 mg/kg (±)-amphetamine responded appropriately for saline when given 0.25 to 1.0 mg/kg (±)-DOM. Winter (1975) trained animals in a one-lever task to discriminate 10 mg/kg mescaline from saline. Response generalization to this dose of mescaline was produced by 0.3 mg/kg (±)-DOM, but not by (+)-amphetamine (0.1 - 1.0 mg/kg) or cocaine (3 - 30 mg/kg). Tilson et al (1975) found that 0.5 mg/kg (−)-DOM (the more active isomer) was insufficient to produce discriminated responding in a two-lever task. Animals trained on 0.75 mg/kg of the (-)-isomer showed generalization to the drug condition when tested with 0.5 and 0.75 mg/kg (+)-amphetamine. Similarly, animals trained on 1.0 mg/kg (+)-amphetamine responded appropriately for the drug condition when tested with 0.5 or 0.75 mg/kg (-)-DOM. In man, DOM has been shown to produce a mild euphoria at subhallucinogenic doses (Snyder et al, 1967; Snyder et al, 1968) and produce "amphetamine-like" stimulation only at doses which are several fold higher than an hallucinogenic dose (Shulgin, 1972). Discrepancies in the animal discrimination data may, therefore, be a reflection of multiple actions of the drug. Nevertheless, Winter's (1975) data show similarity of 0.3 mg/kg racemic DOM to 10 mg/kg mescaline, making it difficult to understand the inability to train rats to discriminate even larger doses of DOM from saline (Huang, 1972; Tilson et al, 1975). In addition, the discrepant findings concerning generalization to amphetamine cannot be readily accounted for. Differences in methodology in the relevant papers make comparisons of results difficult, but appear insufficient to account for the different findings.

Antagonism of stimulant response control

The results of testing a number of neurochemical agents for ability to antagonize response control by stimulants are summarized in Table 4. Briefly stated, no clear role for acetylcholine, norepinephrine or serotonin in stimulant response control has been found. At the doses tested, atropine did not affect responding controlled by amphetamine (Ho and Huang, 1975), cocaine (Ho and McKenna, 1976), or methylphenidate (Silverman and Ho, in preparation). The serotonin antagonists, cinanserin and methysergide, did not affect response control by amphetamine (Ho and Huang, 1975) nor was the serotonin depletor, *p*-chlorophenylalanine, effective in this respect (Schechter and Cook, 1975). Methylphenidate controlled responding was also not antagonized by cinanserin (Silverman and Ho, in preparation). The noradrenergic blocking agents phentolamine, phenoxybenzamine and propranolol, did not block the discriminative property of amphetamine (Ho and Huang, 1975; Schechter and Cook. 1975), cocaine (Ho and McKenna, 1976) or methylphenidate (Silverman and Ho, in preparation). The dopamine-β-hydroxylase inhibitor, disulfiram, did not antagonize amphetamine-induced response control (Schechter and Cook. 1975). On the other hand, effectiveness of antagonists of dopaminergic function in antagonizing the amphetamine stimulus imply a primary role for this amine. Differences in the control exerted by amphetamine and that exerted by cocaine and methylphenidate are suggested by findings with α-methyl-*p*-tyrosine (AMPT) (Table 4). This compound preferentially depletes newly synthesized catecholamines (Weissman et al, 1966). AMPT antagonism of amphetamine, but not cocaine or methylphenidate, response control suggests necessity of intact stores of newly synthesized catecholamines for the amphetamine cue. Reserpine, which acts on the "reserve" pool of catecholamines (Weissman et al, 1966), antagonizes the cocaine and methylphenidate cues. These findings are consistent with actions of AMPT and reserpine on stereotypy and increased motor activity produced by the stimulants. Reserpine has not been tested for its ability to antagonize amphetamine response control, but this seems unlikely since reserpine does not antagonize other amphetamine actions (Scheel-Krüger, 1971; Van Rossum et al, 1962).

Table 4. Antagonism of psychomotor stimulant responding by various neurochemical agents

Training Drug [mg/kg]	Pretreatment Drug Dose Tested [mg/kg]	Dose Producing Antagonism [mg/kg]	References
(+)-Amphetamine [4]	α-Methyl-p-tyrosine [135]	[135]	18
(+)-Amphetamine [1] (0.5)	α-Methyl-p-tyrosine [200]	[200]	14
(+)-Amphetamine [2] (3)	α-Methyl-p-tyrosine [90, 135]	[90, 135]	19
	Haloperidol [0.05, 0.25, 0.5]	[0.25, 0.5]	
	Disulfiram [100, 200]	None	
	Phenoxybenzamine [10]	None	
	Propranolol [20]	None	
	p-Chlorophenylalanine [300]	None	
(+)-Amphetamine [0.8]	α-Methyl-p-tyrosine [250]	[250]	4
	Pimozide [1]	[1]	
	Atropine [1, 2]	None	
	Cinanserin [15]	None	
	Methysergide [4.5]	None	
	Phentolamine [5, 10]	None	
	Propranolol [10, 15]	None	
	Chlorpromazine [4]	None	
Cocaine [10] (5)	Reserpine [2.5]	[2.5]	5
	Pimozide [1]	[1]	
	Phenoxybenzamine [10]	None	
	Phentolamine [10]	None	
	Propranolol [10]	None	
Methylphenidate [3]	Reserpine [1, 2.5]	[2.5]	25
	Haloperidol [0.15, 0.3, 0.5]	[0.3, 0.5]	
	α-Methyl-p-tyrosine [200]	None	
	Atropine [1]	None	
	Cinanserin [15]	None	
	Phenoxybenzamine [10]	None	
	Propranolol [10]	None	

Where two doses are shown for the training drug, antagonists were tested against the dose shown in parentheses.

III. MECHANISM OF STIMULANT RESPONSE CONTROL

Examination of data summarized in Tables 1 through 4 allows rejection of several possible means by which stimulants might be expected to exert discriminative response control. In summary, these are:

1) A nonspecific "drug state" as the basis for stimulant response control is untenable since drugs from other classes do not generalize to stimulants and vice versa. Specificity of response control by drugs belonging to other classes is also documented (Barry, 1974).

2) Primary importance of peripheral effects can be ruled out since derivatives of stimulants with peripheral but not central action do not generalize to centrally active stimulants (Ho and McKenna, 1976; Richards *et al*, 1973).

3) Anorexia alone is insufficient to account for response control since fenfluramine, which shares the anorexic property of stimulants, does not show generalization to amphetamine (Schechter and Rosecrans, 1972).

4) Hyperactivity *per se* is not a necessity for response control by stimulants as demonstrated by generalization of the amphetamine cue by iproniazid plus β-phenethylamine, a treatment which does not produce hyperactivity (Huang and Ho, 1974a).

5) Nonspecific CNS arousal alone does not account for the findings since nikethamide, strychnine and picrotoxin do not generalize to amphetamine (Huang and Ho, 1974b).

The ability of agents which deplete dopamine or block dopamine receptors to antagonize response control by amphetamine, cocaine and methylphenidate suggests that involvement of dopaminergic systems is the common essential feature of their ability to control discriminated responding.

Perhaps the most unexpected finding in these studies is the ability of the β-adrenergic receptor blocker, propranolol, to produce cocaine appropriate responding in animals trained to discriminate this drug from saline (Ho and McKenna, 1976). This result suggests an antagonism of adrenergic systems on dopaminergic systems with blockade of the former resulting in expression of the latter. Further work is required to clarify this and other possibilities.

IV. REFERENCES

1. Barry, H., III,: Classification of drugs according to their discriminable effects in rats. Fed. Proc. __33__: 1814-1824, 1974.

2. Barry, H., III, and Kubena, R. K.: Discriminative stimulus properties of alcohol, marihuana and atropine. *In* Drug Addiction: Experimental Pharmacology, ed. by J. M. Singh, L. H. Miller and H. Lal, pp. 3-16, Futura, New York, 1972.

3. Harris, R. T., and Balster, R. L.: An analysis of the function of drugs in the stimulus control of operant behavior. *In* Stimulus Properties of Drugs, ed. by T. Thompson and R. Pickens, pp. 111-132, Appleton-Century-Crofts, New York, 1971.

4. Ho, B. T., and Huang, J.-T.: Role of dopamine in *d*-amphetamine-induced discriminative responding. Pharmacol. Biochem. Behav. 3: 1085-1092, 1975.

5. Ho, B. T., and McKenna, M. L.: Discriminative stimulus properties of central stimulants. *In* Drug Discrimination and State Dependent Learning, ed. by B. T. Ho, D. Chute and D. W. Richards, III, Academic Press, New York, in press.

6. Huang, J.-T.: Biochemical and pharmacological study of 2,5-dimethoxy-4-methylamphetamine and analogs, Ph.D. dissertation, The University of Texas Graduate School of Biomedical Sciences, Houston, 1972.

7. Huang, J.-T. and Ho, B. T.: The effect of pretreatment with iproniazid on the behavioral activities of β-phenylethylamine in rats. Psychopharmacologia 35: 77-81, 1974a.

8. Huang, J.-T. and Ho, B. T.: Effects of nikethamide, picrotoxin and strychnine on 'amphetamine state'. Eur. J. Pharmacol. 29: 175-178, 1974b.

9. Huang, J.-T. and Ho, B. T.: Discriminative stimulus properties of *d*-amphetamine and related compounds in rats. Pharmacol. Biochem. Behav. 2: 669-673, 1974c.

10. Innes, I. R. and Nickerson, M.: Norepinephrine, epinephrine, and the sympathomimetic amines. *In* The Pharmacological Basis of Therapeutics, ed. by L. S. Goodman and A. Gilman, pp. 477-513, The McMillan Company, New York, 1975.

11. Jones, C. N., Grant, L. D. and Vospalek, D. M.: Temporal parameters of *d*-amphetamine as a discriminative stimulus in the rat. Psychopharmacologia 46: 59-64, 1976.

12. Jones, C. N., Hill, H. F. and Harris, R. T.: Discriminative response control by *d*-amphetamine and related compounds in the rat. Psychopharmacologia 36: 347-356, 1974.

13. Kubena, R. K. and Barry, H., III: Generalization by rats of alcohol and atropine stimulus characteristics to other drugs. Psychopharmacologia 15: 196-206, 1969.

14. Kuhn, D. M., Appel, J. B. and Greenberg, I.: An analysis of some discriminative properties of *d*-amphetamine. Psychopharmacologia 39: 57-66, 1974.

15. Morrison, C. F. and Stephenson, J. A.: Nicotine injections as the conditioned stimulus in discrimination learning. Psychopharmaco-

logia 15: 351-360, 1969.

16. Overton, D. A.: State-dependent learning produced by depressant and atropine-like drugs. Psychopharmacologia 10: 6-31, 1966.

17. Richards, D. W., III, Harris, R. T. and Ho, B. T.: Central control of d-amphetamine-induced discriminative stimuli. Abstract presented at the Third Annual Meeting of the Society of Neurosciences, San Diego, California, Nov. 7-10, p. 340, 1973.

18. Rosecrans, J. A., Goodloe, M. H., Jr., Bennett, G. J. and Hirschhorn, I. D.: Morphine as a discriminative cue: effects of amine depletions and naloxone. Eur. J. Pharmacol. 21: 252-256, 1973.

19. Schechter, M. D. and Cook, P. G.: Dopaminergic mediation of the interoceptive cue produced by d-amphetamine in rats. Psychopharmacologia 42: 185-193, 1975.

20. Schechter, M. D. and Rosecrans, J. A.: Lysergic acid diethylamide (LSD) as a discriminative cue: drugs with similar stimulus properties. Psychopharmacologia 26: 313-316, 1972.

21. Schechter, M. D. and Rosecrans, J. A.: Nicotine as a discriminative cue in rats: inability of related drugs to produce a nicotine-like cueing effect. Psychopharmacologia 27: 379-387, 1972.

22. Schechter, M. D. and Rosecrans, J. A.: d-Amphetamine as a discriminative cue: durgs with similar stimulus properties. Eur. J. Pharmacol. 21: 212-216, 1972.

23. Scheel-Krüger, J.: Comparative studies of various amphetamine analogues demonstrating different interactions with the metabolism of catecholamines in the brain. Eur. J. Pharmacol. 14: 47-59, 1971.

24. Shulgin, A. T.: Stereospecific requirements for hallucinogenesis. J. Pharm. Pharmac. 25: 271-272, 1972.

25. Silverman, P. B. and Ho, B. T.: Manuscript in preparation, 1976.

26. Snyder, S. H., Faillace, L. and Hollister, L.: 2,5-Dimethoxy-4-methylamphetamine (STP): a new hallucinogenic drug. Science 158: 669-670, 1967.

27. Snyder, S. H., Faillace, L. A. and Weingartner, H.: DOM (STP), a new hallucinogenic drug, and DOET: effects in normal subjects. Amer. J. Psychiat. 125: 357-364, 1968.

28. Tilson, H. A., Baker, T. G. and Gylys, J. A.: A comparison of the discriminative stimulus properties of R-2,5-dimethoxy-4-methylamphetamine (R-DOM) and S-amphetamine in the rat. Psychopharmacologia 44: 225-228, 1975.

29. Van Rossum, J. M., Van Der Schoot, J. A. and Hurkmans, J.A.Th.M.:

Mechanism of action of cocaine and amphetamine in the brain. Experientia 18: 229-231, 1962.

30. Waters, W. H., Richards, D. W., III and Harris, R. T.: Discriminative control and generalization of the stimulus properties of D,L-amphetamine in the rat. *In* Drug Addiction: Experimental Pharmacology, Vol. 1, ed. by J. M. Singh, L. Miller, H. Lal, pp. 87-98, Futura, New York, 1972.

31. Winter, J. C.: The effects of 2,5-dimethoxy-4-methylamphetamine (DOM), 2,5-dimethoxy-4-ethylamphetamine (DOET), d-amphetamine, and cocaine in rats trained with mescaline as a discriminative stimulus. Psychopharmacologia 44: 29-32, 1975.

32. Weissman, A., Koe, B. K. and Tenen, S. S.: Antiamphetamine effects following inhibition of tyrosine hydroxylase. J. Pharmacol. Exp. Ther. 151: 339-352, 1966.

DISCRIMINABLE STIMULI PRODUCED
BY MARIHUANA CONSTITUENTS

Edward C. Krimmer and Herbert Barry, III

Department of Pharmacology
University of Pittsburgh
School of Pharmacy
Pittsburgh, Pennsylvania 15261

I. INTRODUCTION

The purpose of the present chapter is to review and summarize studies on the discriminative stimulus attributes of cannabinoids. This group of drugs continues to be the focus of great social and scientific interest. The recent development of techniques for measuring discriminative stimulus attributes of drugs provides a unique criterion for evaluating drug effects in laboratory animals and may be especially valuable for assessing the complex and poorly understood effects of cannabinoids.

II. GENERAL CHARACTERISTICS OF CANNABINOIDS

The term cannabis sativa describes a species of plants composed of more than 100 variations, many of which humans have been familiar with for thousands of years. Products obtained from these plants have been proposed as psychiatric aids, antidepressants, hallucinogens, mood intensifiers, analgesics, treatments for withdrawal symptoms, diuretics, hypotensive agents, hypnotics, stimulants, antibiotics (Hollister, 1971), and the recently proposed use for treatment of glaucoma (National Institute on Drug Abuse, 1975, page 8). Since other more potent drugs are available in each of these areas, cannabis at present appears to have little or no clinical advantage.

The effects of cannabis and cannabis derivatives on animal behavior have been reviewed recently (Miller and Drew, 1974). The chemistry and pharmacology of cannabinoids have also been reviewed (Mechoulam, 1973). Generally there is agreement that high doses of cannabinoids depress various functions. A combination of depressant and stimulant effects has often been reported with lower doses. In measures of spontaneous activity, a period of induced stimulation may precede the depression. Reduced emotionality as measured by decreased defecation was reported by Masur et al. (1971) for THC, but Jarbe and Henriksson (1973b) found elevated vocalization after THC which suggests increased emotionality. Previously Barry and Kubena (1969) showed that the emotional characteristics of animals influence the effect of THC on activity. The same dose decreased activity of animals acclimated to laboratory conditions for five days but increased activity of animals with only one day of acclimation.

The effects of cannabinoids on escape and avoidance behavior seem to suggest that these compounds generally facilitate acquisition of avoidance although there are conflicting reports. Several studies indicate a depressant action on established avoidance and no effect on escape performance (Miller and Drew, 1974).

The effects of THC on aggressive behavior have been equivocal, depending on whether spontaneous, predatory, or irritable aggression is measured (Miczek and Barry, in press). In tests of intraspecies fighting between a dominant and subordinante rat, THC administered to the dominant animal decreased aggressive behavior whereas THC administered to the subordinate rat impaired the defensive-submissive behavior, thereby increasing frequency of biting attacks and number and severity of wounds inflicted (Miczek and Barry, 1974a, 1974b).

Acute and chronic treatments with cannabinoids depress food and water intake and therefore result in loss of body weight (Sofia and Barry, 1974). Elsmore and Fletcher (1972) suggest that this effect may in part be due to learned taste aversions as a result of sickness from high doses of THC.

Tolerance for cannabinoids develops following repeated administration by most routes. Tolerance has been found for several neurophysiological effects of THC and in various behavioral tests in rats measuring sleep, shock avoidance, analgesia, forced motor performance, loss of body weight, and lever pressing for food. Cross tolerance seems to occur between THC and two depressants, pentobarbital and ethanol, during behavioral tests (Paton, 1975).

III. DISCRIMINATION TRAINING WITH CANNABINOIDS

Nearly all human consumption of cannabis products is done in order to achieve some altered mental state as perceived by the individual. Drug discrimination studies provide one possible method to explore the perceived drug effect. They enable us to characterize a drug and to compare it with other drugs by a recently introduced

Table 1

Summary of studies in which rats were trained to discriminate Δ^9-THC from control at 30 min. after i.p. injections, except for 45 min in one study (Hirschhorn and Rosecrans, 1974).

Authors	(mg/kg) i.p.	Percent Correct Δ^9-THC	Control	Task
Kubena & Barry 1972	4	93	92	Single lever, Conflict
Henriksson & Jarbe 1972	5	87	100	T-maze, water escape
	10	100	100	T-maze, water escape
Barry & Kubena 1972	4	93	92	Single lever, Conflict
Jarbe & Henriksson 1973a	5	69		T-maze, water escape
Hirschhorn & Rosecrans 1974	4	75	73	Two lever, food
Jarbe & Henriksson 1974	5	90	*	T-maze, water escape
Barry & Krimmer 1976	2	73	81	Two lever, food
Bueno et al. 1976	5	75	90	T-maze, food

*Data not available

but well verified method (Barry, 1974). A special advantage of this method is that it does not depend on impairment or other disturbance of normal functioning as the measure of the drug effect (Barry and Kubena, 1972).

Characterizations from traditional behavioral tasks are generally similar to those determined in drug discrimination studies, showing for example that depressants resemble other depressants, hypnotics, and sedative, narcotic analgesics resemble other narcotic analgesics, and antimuscarinics resemble other antimuscarinics (Barry, 1974). This type of research appears to have some promise for studying cannabis compounds.

The discriminative properties of a variety of cannabinoids have been reported in a number of studies since the first (Kubena and Barry, 1972). Table 1 summarizes the condition most frequently used with rats, which is Δ^9-THC versus the vehicle or control substance administered intraperitoneally, 30 minutes prior to training. The percentages of correct choices have been taken from the authors' tables or extrapolated from figures when available. The doses of THC (4-5 mg/kg) have been similar in most studies with the exception of a higher dose of 10 mg/kg used by Henriksson and Jarbe (1972) and a lower dose of 2 mg/kg used by Barry and Krimmer (1976).

Percentages of correct choices show that a high level of accuracy was achieved in most of the studies. They do not differ consistently between the drug and nondrug condition. The scores are notably higher in two of three tasks summarized; those are the single-lever conflict and t-maze water-escape tasks. Three of the four studies with slightly lower scores used a food-reward task. One of these (Barry and Krimmer, 1976) also used a lower dose of THC. The unusually poor performance for the T-maze, water-escape task reported by Jarbe and Henriksson (1973a) was obtained during only 12 days of training.

An additional group reported by Henriksson and Jarbe (1972) but not included in Table 1 used THC 5 mg/kg versus vehicle with a series of forced choices under both the drug and vehicle conditions during the early stages of training. The performance reached 100% for both drug and vehicle conditions, slightly better than without forced choice, thereby suggesting some advantage of the forced choice procedure.

Table 2 summarizes studies in which one or more parameters differed from those depicted in Table 1. Jarbe and Henriksson (1974) used hashish, inhaled through the lungs. Smoke produced by burning 2.8 g of hashish was inhaled by groups of 3 rats prior to drug training sessions while chevril smoke was inhaled as the control.

Jarbe and Henriksson (1974) also trained rats to discriminate Δ^8-THC, which is a Δ^9-THC analog, from the nondrug condition. Three separate groups were trained to discriminate Δ^9-THC from atropine, pentobarbital, or phencyclidine. Each group learned the differential response with a high level of accuracy, suggesting that very different effects were perceived for each drug.

The last three studies shown in Table 2 have used species other than rats. Ferraro et al. (1974) administered Δ^9-THC or vehicle orally to three monkeys 2.5 hours prior to discriminative training while Henriksson et al. (1975) trained two pigeons to make discriminative responses 90 minutes after intramuscular injection of Δ^9-THC or vehicle. In the third study gerbils were used by Jarbe et al. (1975b). The task was shock escape in a t-maze with Δ^9-THC (0.5, 2, 8, 12, or 16 mg/kg) being discriminated from vehicle at 30 minutes after i.p. injection. All groups met a learning criterion of eight correct first-trial choices out of ten

Table 2

Summary of studies in which several species were trained to discriminate various cannabinoids (Condition A) from the control or a second drug (Condition B).

Authors, subjects, route, interval & task	Condition A Drug	Dose (mg/kg)	Percent Correct	Condition B Drug	Dose (mg/kg)	Percent Correct
Jarbe & Henriksson 1974 Rats, inhalation Approx. 9 min. T-maze, water escape	Hashish Smoke	2,800	94	Chevril Smoke	0	–
Rats, i.p. 30 min. except as noted T-maze, water escape	Δ^8-THC Δ^9-THC Δ^9-THC Δ^9-THC	5 5 5 5	91 100 100 100	Vehicle Atropine* Pentobarb. Phencyclidine	0 150 12.5 2	– – – –
Ferraro et al. 1974 Monkeys, p.o. 150 min. Two lever, food	Δ^9-THC	3,4	94	Vehicle	0	87
Henriksson et al. 1975 Pigeons, i.m. 90 min. Two lever, food	Δ^9-THC	0.25	96	Vehicle	0	–
Jarbe et al. 1975b Gerbils, i.p. 30 min. T-maze, shock escape	Δ^9-THC Δ^9-THC Δ^9-THC Δ^9-THC Δ^9-THC	0.5 2 8 12 16	– 90 96 – –	Vehicle Vehicle Vehicle Vehicle Vehicle	0 0 0 0 0	– 90 93 – –

* Interval 15 min

– Data not available

---

consecutive sessions but the main emphasis of the report was on the 2 and 8 mg/kg groups, both of which achieved 90% or better correct choices for the drug and nondrug conditions. Generally in each study discriminative response control with cannabinoids has been very good.

Table 3

ED_{50} scores in tests with the specified compounds for the response trained in a discrimination of Δ^9-THC from control.

Test Drug	Training dose (mg/kg)			
	5	5	4	2
Δ^9-THC	1.7	2.7	1.9	0.82
Δ^8-THC	2.6	2.5	–	0.65
11-OH-Δ^9-THC	–	2.5	–	0.36
Marihuana Extracts				
29%	–		–	1.7
17%	–		1.9	–
0.4%	–		0.5	–
Authors and Date	Jarbe & Henriksson (1974)	Bueno et al. (1976)	Kubena & Barry (1972)	Barry & Krimmer (1976)

Several studies provide sufficient data so that ED_{50} scores could be calculated using a procedure described by Barry (1974). Some comparisons of these scores are shown in Table 3. The training conditions in each of the four studies were Δ^9-THC and vehicle. The ED_{50} scores for Δ^9-THC are fairly similar for three studies, using training doses of 4-5 mg/kg. The ED_{50} was notably lower in a fourth study (Barry and Krimmer, 1976) with a lower training dose (2 mg/kg). The ED_{50} shows a fairly constant ratio to the training dose of THC. These ratios, for the four studies listed in Table 3, are .34, .54, .48, and .41 respectively.

The fourth study in addition shows rather low ED_{50} scores for the Δ^8-THC analog and the metabolite, 11-OH-Δ^9-THC. These values are additionally impressive because a food reward task was used and in Table 1 overall performance achieved for the 2-lever food task was slightly lower than that for other studies.

Table 3 also shows that several crude marihuana extracts of various purity have been tested and found to generalize to the drug condition. Comparing the THC content of the marihuana extracts with the same dose of pure THC, the ED_{50} was higher for the marihuana extract with the highest THC content (29%) and lower for the extract with the lowest THC content (0.4%). The ED_{50} for the extract with 17% THC content was equipotent with the same amount of pure THC. These comparisons suggest that some other constituents of marihuana antagonized the THC effect in the most concentrated extract (29% THC) and enhanced the effect of THC in the most dilute extract (0.4% THC). The most concentrated extract excluded water-soluble constituents which might have behavioral effects (Braude and Szara, vol. 2, page 531).

In the study by Jarbe et al. (1975b), shown in Table 2, using gerbils trained with Δ^9-THC, training doses of 2 and 8 mg/kg yielded ED_{50} scores of 0.18 and 0.84 mg/kg respectively. These ratios to the training dose are .09 and .11, respectively. The remarkably low ED_{50} doses and ratios indicate that the gerbil is capable of acquiring strong sensitivity to the stimulus effects of THC. This appears to be a learned sensitivity because the initial rate of learning was generally slower than with pentobarbital in a separate group.

Jarbe and Henriksson (1974) conducted several useful tests with other compounds in two groups shown in Table 2, one trained to discriminate Δ^8-THC from vehicle and the other trained to discriminate hashish from chevril smoke. These authors found that for animals trained to discriminate Δ^8-THC (10 mg/kg) from control, the ED_{50} for this drug was 2.5 mg/kg (.25 ratio to the training dose) and the drug response was elicited by sufficiently high doses of Δ^9-THC (ED_{50} = 5.0 mg/kg). In animals trained to discriminate hashish smoke from control, the drug response was elicited by sufficiently high doses of Δ^9-THC (ED_{50} = 1.4 mg/kg) and Δ^8-THC (ED_{50} < 10.0 mg/kg).

A long and diverse list of compounds that do not elicit the Δ^9-THC response is shown under six broad categories in Table 4. Successive studies have substantiated and extended the conclusion that Δ^9-THC does not resemble a wide variety of depressants, a number of stimulants, hallucinogens, neurotransmitter antagonists, and narcotics or narcotic antagonists.

IV. PHARMACOLOGICAL VARIATIONS

Complete tolerance to the effects of cannabis products has been reported for some animal studies using the rotating rod (Barns and Fried, 1974), shock avoidance (Newman et al., 1974), or pigeons pecking for food (Kosersky et al., 1974). Limited tolerance to physiological effects has been found in humans (Hollister and Tinklenberg, 1973) and the results are even less conclusive for the subjective effects (Rossi et al., 1974).

The decreased sensitivity to drug effects, produced by tolerance, may be expected to impair drug discrimination. Accordingly, Ferraro (1976) has suggested and given evidence that drug discrimination is resistant to tolerance. Bueno and Carlini (1972) first demonstrated the impaired performance for a rope-climbing task produced by administering marihuana extract i.p. to rats. This impairment disappeared following 14 days of chronic treatment with the extract (10 mg/kg), indicating the development of tolerance. These same animals subsequently learned a two-lever food-reward discriminative task at 45 minutes after i.p. injection of the same extract or vehicle. The percentage of correct choices reached 78% with the drug and 79% with the vehicle. An overall lower lever-pressing rate noted during drug sessions early in discrimination training also disappeared with successive training. Although this study did not include a comparison with nontreated animals, the performance is

Table 4

Compounds that elicited the response trained with vehicle or control conditions rather than Δ^9-tetrahydrocannabinol, tested at the indicated dose ranges in the designated studies.

Drug	Dosage range tested mg/kg		Studies tested
	lowest	highest	
Depressants and Sedatives			
Pentobarbital	10	20	1,2,3,4,5,6,7
Phenobarbital	60		3
Alcohol	500	2000	1,2,3,7
Chlordiazepoxide	15		1,2
Diazepam	3.75	7.5	3,4
Chlorpromazine	1	5	1,3,7
Stimulants			
Cocaine	5	20	
Yohimbine	7.5		
Amphetamine	0.5	5	
Nortryptiline	30	5	
Cannabinoids and their Antagonists			
Cannabinol	4	60	1,3,4,5
Cannabidiols	4	150	1,3,4,5,7
Tacrine	2.5	5	3
Phenitrone	15	30	3
Hallucinogens			
Mescaline	15	30	1
LSD-25	0.05	0.2	1,5
Psilocybin	3		
Ditran	0.03	12.5	3,4,5
Phencyclidine	1	2	3,4
DMT	2	4	1
Neurotransmitters: agonist and antagonists			
Atropine	1.25	150	1,3,4,6
Scopolamine	0.25	100	1,3,4
Apomorphine	0.5	2	7

Table 4 Cont'd

Drug	Dosage range tested mg/kg		Studies tested
	lowest	highest	
Narcotics and their Antagonists			
Morphine	4	8	1,3
Levallophan	30	60	3

	Authors	Training drug (dose)
1	Kubena & Barry 1972; Barry & Kubena 1972	Δ^9-THC (4 mg/kg)
2	Barry & Krimmer 1976	Δ^9-THC (2 mg/kg)
3	Jarbe & Henriksson 1974	Δ^9-THC (5 mg/kg)
4	Jarbe & Henriksson 1974	Hashish Smoke (2.8 g)
5	Henriksson, Johansson & Jarbe 1975	Δ^9-THC (0.25 mg/kg)
6	Jarbe, Johansson & Henriksson 1975b	Δ^9-THC (2,8)
7	Bueno, Carlini, Finkelfarb & Suzuki 1976	Δ^9-THC (5 mg/kg)

comparable to other studies using a similar task with Δ^9-THC, shown in Table 1. The drug response by these animals trained with extract was also elicited by Δ^9-THC (5 mg/kg).

The study by Jarbe and Henriksson (1973a), shown in Table 1, included two additional groups, one administered THC (5 mg/kg) and the other vehicle, orally on each of 18 days prior to the start of discrimination training. The percentage of correct choices during the subsequent 12 days of training was 72% for the vehicle group and 56% for the THC group, thereby indicating decreased sensitivity to the cueing effects of THC during 12 days of discrimination training.

Hirschhorn and Rosecrans (1974) used a different technique for studying tolerance. These authors first trained a two-lever food-reward task using Δ^9-THC (4 mg/kg i.p.) or vehicle. After 40 training sessions, additional daily treatment with Δ^9-THC was administered s.c. immediately after the ongoing discriminative training, with progressively increasing doses (8, 16, 32 mg/kg/day). Tolerance to the discriminative effect of Δ^9-THC tested 24 hours afterward, was only partial and was limited to the highest dose (32 mg/kg) given during chronic treatment. The authors acknowledged the possibility that the animals became highly tolerant to THC but compensated, in effect performing a progressively more difficult discrimination.

Attempts to antagonize the discriminative effects of THC have been limited to a study by Jarbe and Henriksson (1974). Animals trained to discriminate Δ^9-THC or hashish smoke from the control conditions were tested with the training drug condition in conjunction with other compounds. The potential antagonists were selected because these authors and other researchers had previously shown that these compounds reversed or altered the effects of THC in other tasks. The list includes chlorpromazine, phenitrone, morphine, diazepam, levallorphan, d-amphetamine, tacrine, cannabinol, and cannabidiol. None of these compounds antagonized the discriminative effects of THC.

The routes of administration of cannabinis products thus far in this review have included intraperitoneal, the most common, and the less frequently used intramuscular, oral, and inhalation. Each produced strong discriminative response control. Jarbe and Henriksson (1974) concluded that the inhalation route is more potent than the intraperitoneal route, but pure Δ^9-THC has not been administered by inhalation. The ED_{50} of 1.4 mg/kg intraperitoneally for Δ^9-THC calculated for their animals trained with hashish smoke in air is similar to ED_{50} scores determined in animals trained with 4-5 mg/kg of Δ^9-THC using the intraperitoneal route in both tests.

Barry and Krimmer (1976) have compared effectiveness of several routes, not including inhalation, in animals trained with Δ^9-THC (2 mg/kg i.p.). These authors found that the ED_{50} score was substantially lower after i.v. administration (0.27 mg/kg) and substantially higher after oral administration (2.9 mg/kg) than after the i.p. administration used in training (0.87 mg/kg). These relative potencies are consistent with usual pharmacological effects. The drug responses elicited through other routes also give evidence for a systemic pharmacological cue for THC rather than a cue produced by local irritation at the injection site.

The temporal parameters of a drug effect are of particular importance in drug discrimination studies because it is desirable to select the training interval at which the drug effect is maximal and stable. These goals are influenced by the dose, route of administration, and to some extent the species involved. No single study has systematically investigated these variables but time functions for four separate reports are compared in Figure 1. Unfortunately each was with a different route, dose, and species. However, all used discrimination of Δ^9-THC from vehicle so that some comparisons can be made. The data for the i.p. route in the top portion of Figure 1 indicate in rats a rapid onset of drug stimulus, within 7.5 minutes. The onset is slightly slower for gerbils and as expected it is considerably more rapid for both species than either the oral or intramuscular route shown in the lower portion of Figure 1 for monkeys and pigeons. The duration of stimulus activity is longest for the p.o. route, tested in monkeys. With each route, the drug stimulus is effective for a fairly prolonged duration.

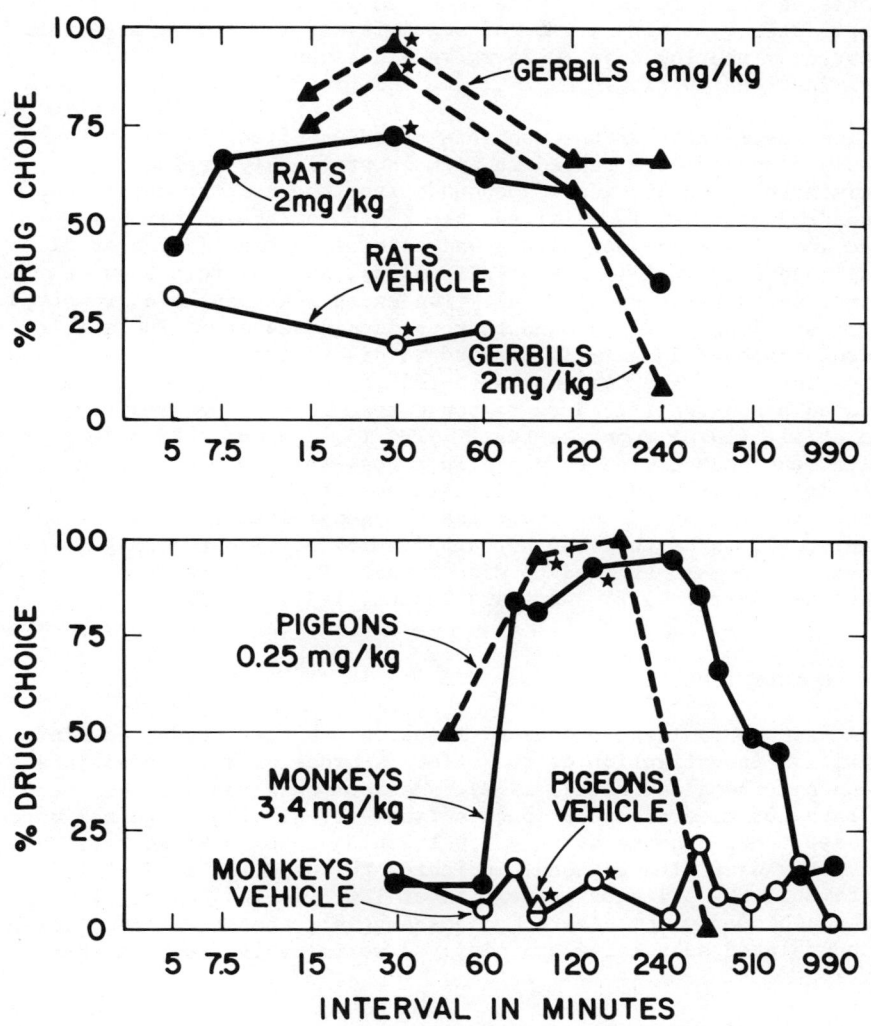

Figure 1. Percentage drug choice made by several species during tests when Δ^9-THC (filled symbols) or vehicle (open symbols) was administered at various times to animals trained to discriminate Δ^9-THC from vehicle. The asterisks indicate the training conditions (30 minutes for rats and gerbils, 90 minutes for pigeons and 150 minutes for monkeys).

The comparisons among routes and time intervals indicate that these variations are not critical for maintaining the discriminative response when a long enough time is given for the drug to reach the site of action. A high degree of sentivity to THC in the pigeon is suggested by the low dose (0.25 mg/kg) that was sufficient for the discriminative learning.

The specificity of the cannabis stimulus effect is evident when cannabis compounds are tested in animals previously trained to discriminate non-cannabinoid compounds from the nondrug condition. The nondrug response is elicited when Δ^9-THC or Δ^8-THC have been tested in animals trained with phencyclidine, ditran (Jarbe et al. 1975a), pentobarbital (Jarbe et al. 1975b), and chlordiazepoxide (Krimmer and Barry, unpublished). Two exceptions have been reported. Cameron and Appel (1973) found that various doses of Δ^9-THC elicited the drug response in animals trained to discriminate LSD from saline. The response to Δ^9-THC was not dose-related and therefore may have indicated a non-specific drug response to a novel drug condition. Bueno et al. (1976) reported that Δ^9-THC (5, 2.5 and 1.25 mg/kg) elicited the amphetamine response in a dose-related manner when tested in rats trained to discriminate amphetamine (1 mg/kg) from saline. In both of these exceptions the generalization was assymetrical, as neither LSD nor amphetamine elicits the drug response in animals trained to discriminate THC from vehicle (Kubena and Barry, 1972; Barry and Kubena, 1972; Henriksson et al., 1975).

V. CONCLUSIONS

A reasonably large amount of research has been conducted since the initial investigation of the stimulus properties of cannabinis compounds (Kubena and Barry, 1972). Most of this research has been with rats but several other species (monkeys, gerbils, pigeons) have also been used. The relatively low training dose (0.25 mg/kg), effectively used with pigeons, indicates this species is especially sensitive to the stimulus properties of THC. A high degree of success achieved with these compounds suggests that the effects of THC and related substances are highly discriminable from the control condition.

The stimulus properties of THC are resistant to tolerance. The i.p. route of administration is most frequently used but the p.o., i.m., i.v., and inhalation routes have also been shown effective after a time interval long enough for the drug to reach the site of action. In accordance with relative rates of absorption and distribution, THC has a more rapid onset for the intraperitoneal route, within 7.5 minutes, than for the oral or intramuscular route. The duration of the discriminative drug stimulus is more than 2 hours by the i.p. and i.m. routes and more than 4 hours by the p.o. route.

ED_{50} scores are slightly less than 50% of the training doses in studies of rats receiving Δ^9-THC i.p., at doses of 5, 4 and 2 mg/kg. The ED_{50} score for pigeons also seems to be about 50% of the training dose. ED_{50} scores of approximately 10% of the training dose, calculated for gerbils, suggest this species can acquire a high degree of sensitivity to the stimulus effects of THC.

Animals trained to discriminate cannabis compounds from the control condition have been tested with a rather long list of diverse compounds, including a wide variety of depressants, a number of stimulants, hallucinogens, neurotransmitter antagonists, narcotic agonists and antagonists, and cannabinoid antagonists. These compounds do not elicit the Δ^9-THC response, indicating that cannabis products are a unique group of compounds that cannot be added to any presently known category.

VI. ACKNOWLEDGEMENTS

Preparation of this paper was supported by NIDA Post-Doctoral Research Fellowship DA-2376 (to E. C. K.), by NIMH Research Scientist Development Award K2-MH-5921 (to H. B.), and by NIMH Research Grant MH-13595 (to both authors).

VII. REFERENCES

Barns, C. and Fried, P. A.: Tolerance to Δ^9-THC in adult rats with differential Δ^9-THC exposure when immature or during early adulthood. Psychopharmacologia 34: 181-190, 1974.

Barry, H., III: Classification of drugs according to their discriminable effects in rats. Fed. Proc. 33: 1814-1824, 1974.

Barry, H., III and Krimmer, E. C.: Discriminative Δ^9-THC stimulus tested with several doses, routes, intervals and a marihuana extract. In Pharmacology of Marihuana, vol. 2, ed. by M. C. Braude and S. Szara, pp. 535-538, Raven, New York, 1976.

Barry, H., III and Kubena, R. K.: Acclimation to laboratory alters response to Δ^1-tetrahydrocannabinol. Proc. 77th Ann. Conv. of the Amer. Psychol. Assoc., 4: 865-866, 1969.

Barry, H., III and Kubena, R. K.: Discriminative stimulus characteristics of alcohol, marihuana and atropine. In Drug Addiction: Experimental Pharmacology, ed. by J. M. Singh, L. Miller and H. Lal, pp. 3-16, Futura Publishing, Mount Kisco, 1972.

Braude, M. C. and Szara, S., Eds.: Pharmacology of Marihuana, 2 vols., Raven, New York, 1976.

Bueno, O. F. A. and Carlini, E. A.: Dissociation of learning in marihuana tolerant rats. Psychopharmacologia 25: 49-56, 1972.

Bueno, O. F. A., Carlini, E. A., Finkelfarb, E. and Suzuki, J. S.: Δ^9-Tetrahydrocannabinol, ethanol, and amphetamine as discriminative stimului-Generalization tests with other drugs. Psychopharmacologia 46: 235-243, 1976.

Cameron, O. G. and Appel, J. B.: A behavioral and pharmacological analysis of some discriminable properties of d-LSD in rats. Psychopharmacologia 33: 117-134, 1973.

Elsmore, T. F. and Fletcher, G. V.: Delta-9 tetrahydrocannabinol: Aversive effects in rat at high doses. Science 175: 911-912, 1972.

Ferraro, D. P.: A behavioral model of marihuana tolerance. In Pharmacology of marihuana, col. 2, ed. by M. C. Braude and S. Szara, pp. 475-486. Raven, New York, 1976.

Ferraro, D. P., Gluck, J. P. and Morrow, C. W.: Temporally-related stimulus properties of Δ^9-Tetrahydrocannabinol in monkeys. Psychopharmacologia 35: 305-316, 1974.

Henriksson, B. G. and Jarbe, T.: Δ^9-Tetrahydrocannabinol used as discriminative stimulus for rats in position learning in a T-shaped water maze. Psychon. Sci. 27: 25-26, 1972.

Henriksson, B. G., Johansson, J. O. and Jarbe, T. U. C.: Δ^9-Tetrahydrocannabinolproduced discrimination in pigeons. Pharmacol. Biochem. and Behav. 3: 771-774, 1975.

Hirschhorn, I. D. and Rosecrans, J. A.: Morphine and Δ^9-Tetrahydrocannabinol: Tolerance to the stimulus effects. Psychopharmacologia 36: 243-253, 1974.

Hollister, L. E.: Marihuana in man: Three years later. Science 172: 21-29, 1971.

Hollister, L. E. and Tinklenberg, J. R.: Subchronic oral doses of marihuana extract. Psychopharmacologia 29: 247-252, 1973.

Jarbe, T. U. C. and Henriksson, B. G.: Open-field behavior and acquisition of discriminative response control in Δ^9-THC tolerant rats. Experientia 29: 1251-1253, 1973a.

Jarbe, T. U. C., Henriksson, B. G.: Vocalization: a characteristic cannabis induced behavior in the rats? Physiol. Psychol. 1: 351-353, 1973b.

Jarbe, T. U. C. and Henriksson, B. G.: Discriminative response control produced with hashish, tetrahydrocannabinols (Δ^8-THC and Δ^9-THC), and other drugs. Psychopharmacologia 40: 1-16, 1974.

Jarbe, T. U. C., Johansson, J. O. and Henriksson, B. G.: Drug discrimination in rats: The effects of phencyclidine and ditran. Psychopharmacologia 42: 33-39, 1975a.

Jarbe, T. U. C., Johansson, J. O. and Henriksson, B. G.: Δ^9-tetrahydrocannabinol and pentobarbital as discriminate cues in the Mongolian gerbil (Meriones unguiculatos). Pharmacol. Biochem. and Behav. 3: 403-410, 1975b.

Kosersky, D. S., McMillan, D. E. and Harris, L. S.: Δ^9-Tetrahydrocannabinol and 11-Hydroxy-Δ^9-Tetrahydrocannabinol: Behavioral effects and tolerance development. J. Pharmacol. Exp. Ther. 189: 61-65, 1974.

Kubena, R. K. and Barry, H., III: Stimulus characteristics of marihuana components. Nature 235: 397-398, 1972.

Masur, J., Martz, R. M. W. and Carlini, E. A.: Effects of acute and chronic administration of cannabis sativa and (-) Δ^9trans-tetrahydrocannabinol on behavior of rats in an open field. Psychopharmacologia 19: 388-397, 1971.

Mechoulam, R.: Marijuana: Chemistry, Pharmacology, Metabolism and Clinical Effects, Academic, New York, 1973.

Miczek, K. A. and Barry, H., III: Effects of Δ^9-tetrahydrocannabinol on aggressive behavior in laboratory rats. In Drug Addiction. Vol. 3: Neurobiology and Influences on Behavior, ed. by I. M. Singh and H. Lal, p 19-38, Stratton International Medical Book Corp., New York, 1974a.

Miczek, K. A. and Barry, H., III: Δ^9-tetrahydrocannabinol and aggressive behavior in rats. Behav. Bio. 11: 261-267, 1974b.

Miczek, K. A. and Barry, H., III: Pharmacology or sex and aggression In Textbook of Behavioral Pharmacology, ed. By S. D. Glick and J. Goldfarb, C. V. Mosby, St. Louis, In Press.

Miller, L. L. and Drew, W. G.: Cannabis: Review of Behavioral effects in animals. Psychological Bul 81: 401-417, 1974.

National Institute of Drug Abuse: Marihuana and Health: Fifth Annual Report. U. S. Government Printing Office, Washington, D. C., 1975.

Newman, L. M., Lutz, M. P. and Domino, E. F.: Δ^9-THC and some CNS depressants: Evidence for cross-tolerance in the rat. Arch. Int. de Pharmacodyn. et de Therap., 207: 254-259, 1974.

Paton, W. D. M.: Pharmacology of Marijuana. In: Annual Review of Pharmacology 15, ed. by H. W. Elliott, R. George and R. Okun, pp. 191-220, 1975.

Rossi, A. M., Babor, T. F., Meyer, R. E. and Mendelson, J. H.: Mood States, In: The use of marihuana: A psychological and physiological inquiry, ed. by J. H. Mendelson, A. M. Rossi and R. E. Meyer, pp. 115-133, Plenum, New York, 1974.

Sofia, R. D. and Barry, H., III: Acute and chronic effects of Δ^9-tetrahydrocannabinol on food intake by rats. Psychopharmacologia 39: 213-222, 1974.

DISCRIMINATIVE STIMULUS PROPERTIES OF HALLUCINOGENS: BEHAVIORAL ASSAY OF DRUG ACTION

Donald M. Kuhn, Francis J. White and James B. Appel

Behavioral Pharmacology Laboratory
Department of Psychology
University of South Carolina
Columbia, S.C. 29208

I. INTRODUCTION

In this chapter we will review existing literature on the discriminative stimulus properties of several drugs which are often classified as hallucinogens. At the same time we will try to answer several questions about the usefulness of this procedure. For example, can it be used as a specific behavioral assay or screening technique for hallucinogens? Can the mechanism of action of hallucinogenic drugs be effectively studied and, if so, can it tell us anything about the nature of hallucinations?

Hallucinogens, for the present purpose, are those compounds which have in common the ability to induce "psychotomimetic"-like effects in humans. While the prototypic drug in this class is lysergic acid diethylamide (LSD), we will also discuss psilocybin, mescaline, ditran, and phencyclidine (PCP). Although almost any drug in large enough doses can induce hallucinations in man, we have simply restricted the scope of our review to include those drugs not covered in extenso elsewhere in this volume. Partial reviews on this subject have appeared previously (Barry, 1974; Winter, 1974a).

II. METHODOLOGICAL CONSIDERATIONS

Any number of experimental procedures have been used to study the discriminative stimulus properties of hallucinogens. The two most frequently studied are shock escape in either a

T-maze or a three compartment box and choice responding for food or water reinforcement in two lever operant chambers [see Overton (1974) for a complete discussion of methodology]. The lever-pressing situation is somewhat more flexible because different schedules of reinforcement can be used to produce different rates of responding. Since response rate is apparently independent of choice, the effects of drugs on both of these variables can be studied simultaneously and thus provide additional information.

Drug discrimination experiments can be classified into two broad categories, transfer and antagonism, each of which involves a specific purpose. In transfer experiments, rats which have been trained to discriminate some drug from placebo are given various "test" compounds to study the degree of similarity (generalization) between training and test (drug) stimuli. With hallucinogens, transfer experiments are often concerned with the hypothesis that drugs which have similar subjective effects in man will also have similar discriminative stimulus properties in rats. In antagonism experiments, attempts are made to block (or in some cases potentiate) a drug cue with treatments which alter the functional activity of transmitter containing neuronal systems. The aim of these studies, of course, is to delineate the mechanisms which mediate the drug cue and, perhaps, additional related properties (i.e. subjective effects in man).

Obviously, before testing of any kind can be accomplished, the drug discrimination must first be established. Existing operant procedures for training drug discriminations are often laborious and time-consuming (see Colpaert et al., 1976). Typically, rats are first trained to lever press; after responding is "appropriate" to the schedule of reinforcement, drug and placebo injections (discriminative stimuli) are given to establish choice responding (left or right lever pressing). By combining these two phases we have found that acquisition of a drug-placebo discrimination can be facilitated at least for some drugs. Thus, on Day 1 of training, water deprived rats are injected with the drug solvent (usually 0.9% NaCl) and shaped to press one lever (the saline lever); the other lever is removed. The initial schedule of reinforcement on Day 1 is FR 1 (i.e., each barpress results in water reinforcement). This schedule is gradually increased to FR 32 throughout Days 1 and 2. On Day 3 rats are injected with the training drug and placed in the operant chamber with only the other (drug) lever present. Pressing the drug lever results in water reinforcement initially on an FR 1 and as before this schedule is rapidly increased from FR1 to FR 32. On Day 4 drug injections are repeated and training continues on the drug lever (FR32). Training progresses on a double alternation sequence until all rats have had the opportunity to respond for 4-6 days on each lever (preceded by appropriate injections). Thereafter, rats are given either drug or placebo and placed in the chambers with both levers present. Responding on the lever appropriate for the substance injected is reinforced on an FR 32 schedule of reinforcement. Responding on the inappropriate lever has no programmed consequences. Discrimination training continues until rats' initial choice (i.e., the 32 responses prior to the first reinforcement) is greater than 90% correct. Using this "errorless" training procedure we have found that rats learn various drug (LSD, pentazocine)-solvent discriminations to a level of 90% correct in 10-15 days. Our procedure might produce even more rapid acquisition if incorrect responding were punished (e.g., resulted in a time-out or foot shock).

Once the drug discrimination is established transfer tests and antagonism studies can be initiated. After treating rats with the test drug of interest we place the animals in the operant chambers and allow responding to continue until 32 responses have been emitted on one lever or the other. The rats are then removed from the apparatus without having been reinforced (extinction). Test data should always be gathered in extinction to avoid confounding subsequent results by allowing additional learning to occur.

III. GENERAL CHARACTERISTICS

Before proceeding to the discussion of data from transfer test and antagonism studies we will briefly describe some general characteristics of the discriminative stimuli produced by hallucinogens. It has been demonstrated for PCP and ditran, at least, that acquisition of a drug discrimination is dose related (Jarbe et al., 1975). The larger doses produce the most rapid acquisition as expected. If the dose is too small, acquisition may be protracted or may not occur at all. Once a drug discrimination is well established tests with various doses of the training drug produce orderly variations in response choice. This is true for LSD (Cameron and Appel, 1973; Hirschhorn and Winter, 1971; Greenberg et al., 1975a) and mescaline (Browne et al., 1974; Browne and Ho, 1975b; Hirschhorn and Winter, 1971). Overton (1974) has pointed out that dose-response gradients for drug discriminability are determined largely by the training dose used to establish the discrimination. Therefore, tests with other doses of the training drug are not dose response functions for discriminability, in a pharmacological sense, because this variable should not be influenced by the training dose. Thus, dose response curves represent relative, not absolute, relationships between the test doses and the training dose. We recently found

that the sensitivity to (or discriminability of) submaximal doses of
LSD could be altered by a behavioral manipulation (Greenberg
et al., 1975a). After completing a dose response study in rats
trained to discriminate 80 ug/kg of LSD from saline, we reinforced
rats for responding on the LSD lever after 10 ug/kg. This dose
originally produced only 30% responding on the LSD lever (in
extinction). It was evident that the rats quickly learned this new
discrimination; lever choice after 10 ug/kg of LSD reached over
80% after just eight injections of this lower dose. We then
returned the rats to the original discrimination (80 ug/kg LSD vs.
saline) and re-determined the dose response curve. These data
are presented in Fig. 1. We found that the dose response curve
was shifted to the left as a result of reinforcing rats at the lower
dose of LSD. These data point out the importance of the training
dose in determining subsequent dose response relationships. In
addition, our results with these extremely low doses of LSD point
to the sensitivity and flexibility of the drug discrimination procedure.

Another important variable in behavioral pharmacological
experiments is tolerance, defined as the diminution in a (behavioral) response to a drug after repeated administration of that
drug. Tolerance to the stimulus properties of hallucinogens has
not been extensively studied. A dosage regimen of LSD (acute
tolerance) which produces tolerance to the disruptive effects of
LSD (Freedman et al., 1964) does not produce tolerance to the
LSD stimulus (Cameron and Appel, 1973). Winter (1974a) observed
that a mescaline-saline discrimination was not disrupted if LSD
was administered after each saline session. In view of the data
we just presented (Fig. 1), it may be difficult to demonstrate
tolerance to the stimulus properties of a drug. Repeated drug
injections may indeed result in a reduced effect (tolerance) but
the animals' ability to discriminate may not decrease because
they are learning to discriminate smaller doses of the training
drug. Additional studies are needed to assess tolerance to drug
stimulus properties.

IV. RESULTS

A. Transfer Tests with Hallucinogens

The results of transfer tests with hallucinogens are presented
in Tables 1 and 2. LSD can exert control over choice responding under a variety of experimental conditions (Cameron and
Appel, 1973; Hirschhorn and Rosecrans, 1974, 1976; Hirschhorn
and Winter, 1971, 1975; Schechter and Rosecrans, 1972) at extremely low doses (0.01 mg/kg in rats (Greenberg et al., 1975a).
It is typically found that other indole amine hallucinogens such as
psilocybin and phenylethylamine hallucinogens such as

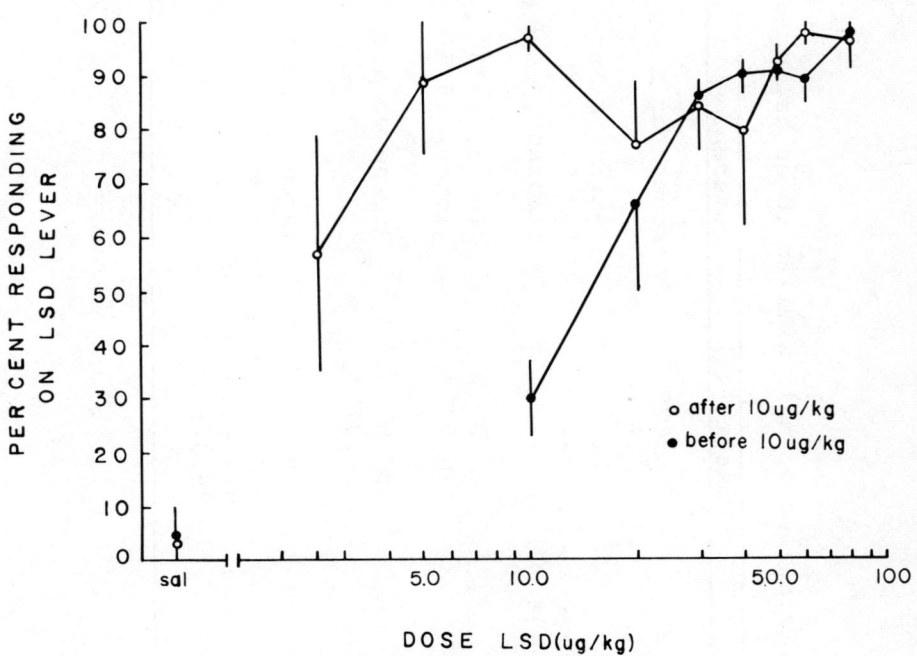

Fig. 1. Per cent of total responding on the LSD lever after various doses of LSD (log scale). Solid circles represent lever choice before the rats were trained to discriminate 10 ug/kg of LSD; open circles represent redetermination of the dose response curve after reinforcing the rats for responding on the LSD lever after 10 ug/kg of LSD. Vertical lines represent ± S.D. All injections were administered 30 min before testing in extinction for lever choice. Each data point is the average of three replications of each dose for 6 animals. (Reproduced with the permission of Psychopharmacology)

Table 1. Drugs which produce discriminative stimuli similar to an hallucinogen

Training	Dose (mg/kg)	Testing	Dose (mg/kg)	Reference
LSD	0.048	Mescaline	22.3, 29.7	Schechter & Rosecrans, 1972
	"	Psilocybin	2.5	"
	0.08	Mescaline	8.0	Cameron & Appel, 1973
	"	Scopolamine	4.0	"
	0.10	Cyclazocine	1.0	Hirschhorn & Rosecrans, 1976
Mescaline	10.0	TMPEA	10.0	Winter, 1973
	"	DOM	0.03	Winter, 1975
	"	DOET	0.03	"
	25.0	DMM	50.0	Browne et al., 1975
	"	Mescaline	0.075*	"
Ditran	3.125, 6.25	Atropine	25.0	Jarbe et al., 1975
PCP	1.0–2.0	Cyclohexamine	0.75–1.0	"
	2.0–6.0	Ketamine	25.0–35.0	"

*Injected intraventricularly

Table 2. Drugs which do not produce discriminative stimuli similar to an hallucinogen

Training	Dose (mg/kg)	Testing	Dose (mg/kg)	Reference
LSD	0.028	Barbital	20.0-160.0	Hirschhorn & Winter, 1975
	0.048	d-amphetamine	2.0,4.0	Schechter & Rosecrans, 1972
	0.072	Morphine	5.0-20.0	Hirschhorn & Rosecrans, 1974
	0.08	Chlorpromazine	0.5	Cameron & Appel, 1973
	"	d-amphetamine	1.0	"
	0.10	Methadone	1.0-6.0	Hirschhorn & Rosecrans, 1976
	"	Meperidine	5.0-10.0	"
	"	Pentazocine	5.0-20.0	"
	"	Nalorphine	1.0-40.0	"
Ditran	3.125,6.25	PCP	2.0-4.0	Jarbe et al., 1975
	"	Δ_9-THC	5.0	"
Mescaline	10.0	DMPEA	10.0-30.0	Winter, 1974b
	"	d-amphetamine	0.1-1.0	Winter, 1975
	"	Cocaine	3.0-30.0	"
	25.0	NMM	10.0-50.0	Browne et al., 1974
	"	NMM	0.025-0.20*	"
	"	TMPA	25.0	Browne & Ho, 1975a
	"	TMPE	25.0-50.0	"
	"	N-acetylmescaline	50.0	"
PCP	2.0-6.0	Ditran	6.25	Jarbe et al., 1975
	"	Δ_8-THC	5.0	"
	"	Δ_8-THC	10.0	"
	"	Pentobarbital	12.5-18.75	"
	"	Morphine	10.0	"
	"	Chlorpromazine	5.0	"

*Injected intraventricularly

mescaline generalize to the LSD stimulus cue (Cameron and Appel, 1973; Hirschhorn and Winter, 1971; Schechter and Rosecrans, 1972). The dysphorigenic narcotic antagonist cyclazocine partially transfers to LSD but nalorphine, which is pharmacologically and subjectively similar to cyclazocine in man (Haertzen, 1970), does not (Hirschhorn and Rosecrans, 1976). There are reports that the cholinolytic agent, ditran, and the dissociative anesthetic, PCP, are psychotomimetic in man (Hollister, 1964; Ketchum et al., 1973). Thus we gave both of these drugs to rats trained to discriminate 0.08 mg/kg LSD from saline. The results are presented in Table 3.

Table 3. Results of transfer test and antagonism studies in rats (N= 12) trained to discriminate 0.08 mg/kg of LSD from saline.

Treatment (mg/kg)	% Responding on LSD Lever
LSD	94.2
saline	4.3
Ditran (1.0)	40.0
(3.0)	26.1
PCP (1.0-4.0)	10.0
Quipazine (2.5)	81.0
LSD + MTP (0.10)	61.2
+ MTP (0.25)	67.2
+ MTP (0.50)	56.0
+ MTP (1.00)	21.7
LSD + HAL (0.50)	93.6
+ HAL (1.00)	95.4

LSD, saline, ditran, and PCP were injected 15 min prior to testing rats for lever choice in extinction. Methiothepin (MTP) and haloperidol (HAL) were given 1 hr before LSD. Quipazine was given 30 min prior to testing for transfer.

Ditran results in a partial transfer to LSD whereas PCP does not. It is interesting that Cameron and Appel (1973) found that scopolamine partially transfers to LSD. We also tested our rats with quipazine, a putative, direct serotonin receptor agonist (Hong et al., 1969), and observed an almost complete transfer to LSD (Table 3). A large variety of compounds do not transfer to LSD; these are listed in Table 2.

While little research has been done with other indole amine

hallucinogens, it has been determined that psilocybin has discriminable properties of its own (Greenberg et al., 1975b; Harris and Balster, 1971).

Numerous studies have established that mescaline has potent discriminative stimulus properties (Hirschhorn and Winter, 1971; Browne et al., 1974; Browne and Ho, 1975 a, b,; Winter, 1973, 1974b, 1975). Much of this research has been devoted to determining if the discriminable cue produced by mescaline is due to mescaline itself or to a structural isomer or metabolite of the parent compound. The stimulus properties of mescaline (3,4,5-trimethoxyphenylethylamine) have been compared to those of its non-hallucinogenic congeners 2,3,4-trimethoxyphenylethylamine (TMPEA) and 3,4-dimethoxyphenyl-ethylamine (DMPEA). TMPEA was shown to produce a discriminable cue and to mimic mescaline (Winter, 1973). However, DMPEA could neither control differential behavior nor mimic the mescaline cue (Winter, 1974b).

Studies with various metabolites of mescaline have determined that the stimulus properties of mescaline reside in the parent compound. Browne et al., (1974) compared N-methylated derivatives of mescaline to mescaline. They found that N-methyl-mescaline (NMM) did not mimic mescaline whereas N, N-dimethyl-mescaline (DMM) did. Since the doses of DMM required to mimic mescaline were twice as large as the dose of mescaline used for training, the authors concluded that an N-methylated metabolite of mescaline probably does not produce the discriminable cue. Additional studies from the same laboratory (Browne and Ho, 1975a) have more clearly established that the mescaline cue is not mediated by a metabolite. This was accomplished by administering various deaminated and N-acetylated mescaline metabolites to rats discriminating mescaline from saline as well as by inhibiting the enzymes involved in the deamination pathway. The results indicated that the metabolites 3,4,5-trimethoxyphenylethanol (TMPE) 3,4,5-trimethoxyphenylacetaldehyde (TMPA), and N-acetyl-mescaline did not mimic mescaline. Inhibition of either aldehyde dehydrogenase or monoamine oxidase potentiated the mescaline cue (Browne and Ho, 1975a).

In a recent study, Winter (1976) demonstrated that the ring substituted amphetamines 2,5-dimethoxy-4-methylamphetamine (DOM) and 2,5-dimethoxy-4-ethylamphetamine (DOET) mimic mescaline whereas d-amphetamine and cocaine do not. While DOM is hallucinogenic in man, DOET is not (Snyder et al., 1968, 1974).

Ditran and PCP are discriminable from saline and from each other (Jarbe et al., 1975). Transfer tests have established that the anticholingeric atropine transfers to ditran whereas PCP and

Table 4. Drugs which antagonize the discriminative stimuli of hallucinogens

Training	Dose (mg/kg)	Antagonist	Dose (mg/kg)	Reference
Mescaline	15.0	Cinanserin	15.0	Browne & Ho, 1975b
	"	Methysergide	5.0	"
	"	Cyproheptadine	5.0	"
Ditran	1.6	Tacrine	5.0	Jarbe et al., 1975
	"	Physostigmine	0.5-1.0	"

Table 5. Drugs which do not antagonize the discriminative stimuli of hallucinogens

Training	Dose (mg/kg)	Testing	Dose (mg/kg)	Reference
LSD	0.072	Methysergide	3.0-10.0	Hirschhorn & Rosecrans, 1972
	"	Cyproheptadine	3.0	"
	"	Atropine	0.5-2.0	"
	"	Naloxone	0.1-0.4	"
	0.08	Chlorpromazine	0.5	Cameron & Appel, 1973
Mescaline	15.0	Xylamidine	1.0	Browne & Ho, 1975b
	"	Atropine	not reported	"
	"	Phentolamine	"	"
	"	Propranolol	"	"
	"	Amphetamine	"	"
	"	Strychnine	"	"
	"	Pimozide	"	"
	"	Picrotoxin	"	"
Ditran	1.6	Yohimbine	5.0	Jarbe et al., 1975
	"	Neostigmine	0.4	"
PCP	2.0	PCPA	310.0	"
	2.0-6.0	TBZ + IMI*	10+2.5, 20+5.0	"

*Tetrabenazine + Imiprimine

Δ^8THC did not (Table 1B). A variety of compounds were also tested for transfer to PCP. Only the structurally related agents ketamine and cyclohexamine mimicked PCP (Jarbe et al., 1975).

B. Antagonism Studies with Hallucinogens

Only limited data are available on the ability of various compounds to attenuate the stimulus properties of hallucinogens. These results are summarized in Tables 4 and 5. Attempts to block the LSD cue with the putative serotonin receptor antagonists cyproheptadine and methysergide, with the anticholinergic atropine, and with the narcotic antagonist naloxone were unsuccessful (Hirschhorn and Rosecrans, 1974). However, we have recently observed a dose related blockade of the LSD stimulus cue following pretreatment with the neuroleptic methiothepin. These data are also included in Table 3. Interestingly, methiothepin displaces LSD from the recently identified LSD receptor (Lovell and Freedman, 1976). We were unable to block LSD with the dopamine receptor antagonist haloperidol.

The stimulus properties of mescaline can be blocked by cinanserin, methysergide, and cyproheptadine; the peripheral serotonin antagonist xylamidine tosylate is without effect (Browne and Ho, 1975b). Depletion of brain serotonin with the tryptophan hydroxylase inhibitor p-chlorophenylalanine (PCPA) potentiates the stimulus properties of submaximal doses of both LSD (Cameron and Appel, 1973) and mescaline (Browne and Ho, 1975b).

Antagonism studies have also been carried out with ditran and PCP. The stimulus cue produced by ditran was blocked by the anticholinesterase agents tacrine and physostigmine, but was unaffected by yohimbine and neostigmine (Jarbe et al., 1975). The discriminative stimulus produced by PCP was neither disrupted by PCPA pretreatment nor blocked by a combination of tetrabenazine and imiprimine which effectively blocks other effects of PCP in rats (Tonge and Leonard, 1972).

V. DISCUSSION

A. Transfer Tests

As mentioned earlier, transfer tests have been carried out in an effort to determine if drugs which have similar subjective effects in man have similar stimulus properties in rats. It was hoped that whatever property causes a drug to be hallucinogenic in man would be the property which makes the same drug discriminable in rats so that the discriminable properties in rats could serve as a useful animal model for predicting and analyzing hallucinogens. Apparently, this has not proven to be the case. For example, TMPEA and DOET, which are not hallucinogenic, transfer to mescaline; cyclazocine, which is subjectively differentiable from LSD in humans, partially transfers to LSD in rats but nalorphine and pentazocine do not; quipazine transfers to LSD but, unfortunately, little is known about its subjective effects in man. Indeed, it seems clear that the drugs presently discussed as hallucinogens are even quite different in terms of their discriminative stimulus properties.

While the behavioral procedure we have been considering may not be an accurate assay of the ability of compounds to induce hallucinations, it does have the capability to detect very subtle features of drugs (structural, resonance form) upon which discriminable similarity is apparently based. For example, only the structurally related drugs ketamine and cyclohexamine transfer to PCP. Thus, the drug discrimination procedure could be used to screen compounds for similarity specifically to LSD, specifically to mescaline etc. Whatever structural variables make such drugs discriminably similar in rats may be necessary to cause similar subjective effects in man but they are not sufficient. We must realize that the task of devising a behavioral assay which is specific for hallucinogens is complicated from the outset by our lack of knowledge of what hallucinations are and the variability inherent in subjective reports of drug effects in man. Indeed, while LSD, mescaline, psilocybin, ditran, and PCP are all reported to induce hallucinations, an LSD hallucination must certainly be different from a ditran or a PCP hallucination. Thus, the usefulness of this procedure is not diminished because it is not a specific assay for hallucinogens. No procedure is. It is, however, one of few behavioral procedures which is sensitive and specific enough to distinguish differences among the various "hallucinogens". Hopefully, subsequent transfer studies will concentrate on structure-activity relationships to determine those features of drugs which make them discriminably similar.

B. Antagonism Studies

The purpose of antagonism studies has been to delineate the mechanism(s) of drug discriminative cues. For some time now the actions of LSD have been attributed to its direct interaction with the central serotonergic neuronal system (Aghajanian, 1972). The results of an interesting transfer experiment suggest that a postsynaptic serotonin receptor is involved. Hirschhorn et al., (1975) trained rats to discriminate midbrain raphe stimulation from non-stimulation. When injected with LSD their rats responded (lever choice) as if they had been stimulated (Hirschhorn et al., 1975). The quipazine transfer to LSD which we observed

(Table 2) also suggests a serotonergic involvement in the LSD cue. It is not clear to us why the LSD cue was not blocked by the serotonin antagonists cyproheptadine and methysergide (Hirschhorn and Rosecrans, 1974). We have found that these agents do in fact block LSD (unpublished observations). Preliminary evidence from our laboratory suggests, furthermore, that it might be more accurate to attribute the mediation of the stimulus properties of LSD to an LSD (rather than a serotonin) receptor. Methiothepin blocks both the LSD stimulus cue and the recently identified d-LSD receptor (Lovell and Freedman, 1976). Methiothepin and haloperidol are approximately equipotent as dopamine receptor antagonists but at doses equimolar to those of methiothepin, haloperidol does not block the LSD cue.

By virtue of the ability of cinanserin, methysergide, and cyproheptadine to block the mescaline cue, it has been concluded that mescaline exerts its cue by stimulating serotonin receptors (Browne and Ho, 1975b). A central locus for the mescaline stimulus was indicated with the demonstration that intraventricularly administered mescaline transfers in a dose related manner to systemically injected mescaline (Browne et al., 1974).

The stimulus properties of ditran are apparently related to the anticholinergic properties of this compound. The anticholinesterase agents tacrine and physostigmine reverse the ditran cue. Since the peripherally acting neostigmine did not block ditran, a central locus of action is also inferred for the stimulus properties of this drug (Jarbe et al., 1975). Little is known about the mechanisms underlying the PCP stimulus cue. The lack of effect of PCPA on the PCP cue is not sufficient to rule out a role for serotonin because PCP may act directly and independently of an intact serotonin system.

Existing data from antagonism studies indicates that the various hallucinogens may also have different mechanisms of action. There is too little data, however, to draw any conclusions. Interpretation of antagonism studies are further complicated by the lack of knowledge of how and where in the brain many of the drugs typically used as antagonists act. Nevertheless, this procedure is ideally suited to study drug mechanisms of action because of its sensitivity and specificity.

VI. CONCLUSIONS

Drugs capable of inducing hallucinations in man can serve as discriminative stimuli in rats. While drugs which are subjectively similar in man will almost certainly have similar discriminative properties in rats, it does not follow that drugs with similar stimulus properties in rats will be subjectively similar in man. Thus, the hallucinogenic liability of a drug cannot be accurately predicted from transfer tests. Antagonism studies appear to offer some very interesting results but the hallucinogens have not yet been studied extensively enough to be able to accurately assess its usefulness in studying drug mechanisms of action. Obviously, tests with other hallucinogens such as dimethyltryptamine or bufotenine are needed.

VII. ACKNOWLEDGEMENTS

Preparation of this manuscript and some of the research described therein was supported by USPHS Research Grants MH-24,333 and MH-24,593 from the National Institute of Mental Health.

VIII. REFERENCES

Aghajanian, G.K.: LSD and CNS transmission. Ann. Rev. Pharmacol. 12: 157-168, 1972.

Barry, H., III.: Classification of drugs according to their discriminable effects in rats. Fed. Proc. 33: 1814-1824, 1974.

Browne, R.G., Harris, R.T., and Ho, B.T.: Stimulus properties of mescaline and N-methylated derivatives: difference in peripheral and direct central administration. Psychopharmacologia (Berl.) 34: 43-56, 1974.

Browne, R.G. and Ho, B.T.: Discriminative stimulus properties of mescaline: mescaline or metabolite? Pharmacol. Biochem. Behav. 3: 109-114, 1975a.

Browne, R.G. and Ho, B.T.: Role of serotonin in the discriminative stimulus properties of mescaline. Pharmacol. Biochem. Behav. 3: 429-435, 1975b.

Cameron, O.G. and Appel, J.B.: A behavioral and pharmacological analysis of some discriminable properties of d-LSD in rats. Psychopharmacologia (Berl.) 33: 117-134, 1973.

Colpaert, F.C., Niemegeers, C.J.E., and Janssen, P.A.J.: Theoretical and methodological considerations on drug discrimination learning. Psychopharmacologia (Berl.) 46: 169-177, 1976.

Freedman, D.X., Appel, J.B., Hartman, F.R., and Molliver, M.E.: Tolerance to behavioral effects of LSD-25 in rats. J.

Pharmacol. exp. Ther. 143: 309-313, 1964.

Greenberg, I., Kuhn, D.M., and Appel, J.B.: Behaviorally induced sensitivity to the discriminable properties of LSD. Psychopharmacologia (Berl.) 43: 229-232, 1975a.

Greenberg, I., Kuhn, D.M., and Appel, J.B.: Comparison of the discriminative stimulus properties of ^{9}THC and psilocybin in rats. Pharmacol. Biochem. Behav. 3: 931-934, 1975b.

Haertzen, C.A.: Subjective effects of the narcotic antagonists cyclazocine and nalorphine on the Addiction Research Center Inventory (ARCI). Psychopharmacologia (Berl.) 18: 366-377, 1970.

Harris, R.T. and Balster, R.L.: An analysis of the function of drugs in the stimulus control of operant behavior. In Stimulus Properties of Drugs, ed. by T. Thompson and R. Pickens, pp. 111-132, 1971.

Hirschhorn, I.D., Hayes, R.L., and Rosecrans, J.A.: Discriminative control of behavior by electrical stimulation of the dorsal raphe nucleus: generalization to lysergic acid diethylamide (LSD). Brain Res. 86: 134-138, 1975.

Hirschhorn, I.D. and Rosecrans, J.A.: A comparison of the stimulus effects of morphine and lysergic acid diethylamide (LSD). Pharmacol. Biochem. Behav. 2: 361-366, 1974.

Hirschhorn, I.D. and Rosecrans, J.A.: Generalization of morphine and lysergic acid diethylamide (LSD) stimulus properties to narcotic analgesics. Psychopharmacology 47: 65-69, 1976.

Hirschhorn, I.D. and Winter, J.C.: Mescaline and lysergic acid diethylamide (LSD) as discriminative stimuli. Psychopharmacologia (Berl.) 22: 64-71, 1971.

Hirschhorn, I.D. and Winter, J.C.: Differences in the stimulus properties of barbital and hallucinogens. Pharmacol. Biochem. Behav. 3: 343-347, 1975.

Hollister, L.E.: Chemical psychosis. Ann. Rev. Med. 15: 203-214, 1964.

Hong, E., Sancillo, L.F., Vargas, R., and Pardo, E.G.: Similarities between the pharmacological actions of quipazine and serotonin. Life Sci. 6: 274-280, 1969.

Jarbe, T.U.C., Johansson, J.O., and Henriksson, B.G.: Drug discrimination in rats: the effects of phencyclidine and ditran. Psychopharmacologia (Berl.) 42: 33-39, 1975.

Ketchem, J.S., Sidell, F.R., Crowell, E.B., Jr., Aghajanian, G.K., and Hayes, A.H., Jr.: Atropine, scopolomine, and ditran: comparative pharmacology and antagonists in man. Psychopharmacologia (Berl.) 28: 121-145, 1973.

Lovell, R.A. and Freedman, D.X.: Stereospecific receptor site for d-lysergic acid diethylamide in rat brain: effects of neurotransmitters, amine antagonists and other psychotropic drugs. Mol. Pharmacol. 12: 620-630, 1976.

Overton, D.A.: Experimental methods for the study of state dependent learning. Fed. Proc. 33: 1800-1813, 1974.

Schechter, M.D. and Rosecrans, J.A.: Lysergic acid diethylamide (LSD) as a discriminative cue: drugs with similar stimulus properties. Psychopharmacologia (Berl.) 26: 313-316, 1972.

Snyder, S.H., Faillace, L.A., and Weingartner, H.: DOM (STP), a new hallucinogenic drug, and DOET; effects in normal subjects. Amer. J. Psychiat. 125: 357-364, 1968.

Snyder, S.H., Ungar, S., Blatchley, R., and Barfknecht, C.F.: Stereospecific actions of DOET (2,5-dimethoxy-4-ethylamphetamine) in man. Arch. Gen. Psychiat. 31: 103-106, 1974.

Tonge, S.R. and Leonard, B.E.: Partial antagonism of the behavioral and neurochemical effects of phencyclidine by drugs affecting monoamine metabolism. Psychopharmacologia (Berl.) 24: 516-520, 1972.

Winter, J.C.: A comparison of the stimulus properties of mescaline and 2,3,4-trimethoxyphenylethylamine. J. Pharmacol. exp. Ther. 185: 101-107, 1973.

Winter, J.C.: Hallucinogens as discriminative stimuli. Fed. Proc. 33: 1825-1832, 1974a.

Winter, J.C.: The effects of 3,4-dimethoxyphenylethylamine in rats trained with mescaline as a discriminative stimulus. J. Pharmacol. exp. Ther. 189: 741-747, 1974b.

Winter, J.C.: The effects of 2,5-dimethoxy-4-methylamphetamine (DOM), 2,5-dimethoxy-4-ethylamphetamine (DOET), d-amphetamine, and cocaine in rats trained with mescaline as a discriminative stimulus. Psychopharmacologia (Berl.) 44: 29-32, 1975.

CHOLINERGIC AND NON-CHOLINERGIC ASPECTS OF THE
DISCRIMINATIVE STIMULUS PROPERTIES OF NICOTINE

John A. Rosecrans and William T. Chance

Department of Pharmacology
Medical College of Virginia
Virginia Commonwealth University
Richmond, Virginia 23298

I. INTRODUCTION

Nicotine is one of the most interesting drugs used by man. Millions of humans (approximately 60 million in the USA) use and have used this drug via tobacco, but its mechanism of reinforcement has yet to be elucidated. Although nicotine, unlike morphine and cocaine, does not reinforce behavior in sub-human species, it does appear to be quite reinforcing in man. Behavioral effects associated with the use of nicotine have not been clearly documented in humans. In animals, however, the drug produces a variety of effects dependent upon baseline behaviors prior to drug administration. Thus, if baseline behaviors are low, nicotine increases these rates whereas a decrease is observed if the baseline behavior rate is initially high. None of these actions of nicotine have been reported in humans, however, and there is still little evidence indicating how the drug is affecting human behavior.

A major research effort in our laboratory has been to determine the mechanisms of action of nicotine upon the brain with the objective of determining why nicotine produces a positive behavioral effect in man. This objective is, however, confounded by several factors not directly related to the effect of nicotine upon the CNS. Since it is not clear as to whether all humans use tobacco because of the presence of nicotine, other factors such as tobacco taste, the operant aspects of smoking, social behavior, peer pressure, etc. must also be considered as motivators of tobacco use. In this discussion, however, we will be focusing on the behavioral effects of nicotine. Whether these effects are expressed as primary or secondary reinforcement is still open to much debate.

Nicotine has long been known to have a specific stimulating effect on peripheral autonomic nervous system preganglionic synapses (nicotinic receptor sites). Excitation of these nicotinic synapses has been shown to elicit the release of acetylcholine (ACh) at postganglionic parasympathetic synapses (muscarinic sites) and norepinephrine (NE) at postganglionic sympathetic synapses (adrenergic sites). In addition, the release of ACh at preganglionic neurons has been observed to produce a nicotine-like response, indicating that nicotine is a cholinomimetic compound. Therefore, there are at least two types of cholinergic receptors which can further be differentiated by the specific antagonists atropine (muscarinic blocker) and hexamethonium (nicotinic blocker). Generalizing these considerations to the CNS, one may hypothesize that nicotine is affecting the brain through any of three mechanisms: (1) directly at a nicotinic receptor site (n-cholinergic), (2) indirectly by the release of ACh at a muscarinic receptor site (m-cholinergic), or (3) indirectly by releasing NE at an adrenergic receptor.

Domino and co-workers (1967) were the first to investigate at which central site nicotine was acting by studying nicotine-induced EEG arousal across several species. This research indicates that the nicotine-produced arousal was associated with a specific nicotinic receptor and was not blocked by the m-cholinergic antagonist, atropine. The centrally-acting n-cholinergic antagonist, mecamylamine, was also shown to completely block the nicotine-induced EEG effects. The central action of nicotine was further elucidated by showing that the EEG arousal was not blocked by hexamethonium, an n-cholinergic antagonist unable to cross the blood-brain barrier because of its quarternary structure. An analogous series of investigations were also conducted with the m-cholinergic agonist, arecoline. These studies established the existence of two separate cholinergic receptors within the CNS which may mediate different behaviors. These receptors are not interconnected (in series) as in the peripheral autonomic nervous system, and may have separate (in parallel) anatomical arrangements in the brain. Thus, there are at least two distinct and separate cholinergic receptors in the CNS by which centrally-acting cholinergic agonists and antagonists can produce behavioral effects.

As previously stated, the behavioral effect of nicotine depended in part upon the baseline behavior prior to the administration of the drug. Bovet and co-workers (1967) were the first to observe this phenomenon in rats, reporting that both high and low rates of behavior were reversed subsequent to drug application. We initiated similar experiments directed toward a determination of the neurochemical bases of these modulating effects upon baseline behaviors. Since serotonin (5-HT)-depleting midbrain raphe lesions have been reported to increase activity levels (Kostowski et al., 1969), we hypothesized that nicotine produced a normalizing (homeostatic) effect on behavior via a cholinergic-serotonergic interaction (Rosecrans, 1971a). It was anticipated that evidence of this interaction could be useful in explaining the positive reinforcing effects of nicotine in humans. In this study, animals were initially separated into high and low activity groups, and both the behavioral and neurochemical effects of nicotine were evaluated. The results of this and several additional experiments (Rosecrans, 1971b; 1972; Rosecrans and Schechter, 1972) indicated that nicotine tended to equalize the activity differences between groups across both strain and sex differences in behavior. Evaluation of the neurochemical data suggested that the baseline activity rates were related to 5-HT levels, but there was no evidence that nicotine was specifically affecting the indoleamine system to yield the observed changes in activity.

While these results appear useful in our attempts to explain some of the behavioral effects of nicotine in humans, our inability to exert control over such behavior or predict these effects have caused difficulty in the design of studies which could elucidate how and where this drug is affecting the brain. These problems necessitated the use of approaches which would meet the necessary criteria of studying the mechanism of the behavioral effects of the drug. Foremost among these criteria was the need of an experimental paradigm that allowed an experimental subject to identify in an objective fashion whether or not nicotine had been administered rather than one which studied the disruptive or excitatory effects of the drug. Evidence toward the establishment of this criterion was provided by a series of experiments designed to study how nicotine affected habituation in rats selected for differences in activity levels (Fig. 1). In this study, low activity subjects habituated (as measured by the increase in activity after the initial exposure) at a faster rate than high activity subjects. These differences in habituation were reversed by the administration of 400 µg/kg of nicotine during the initial exposure to the novel apparatus. The importance of this study was not that nicotine could change habituation rates, but was related to the fact that a single dose of nicotine affected behavior in subsequent test sessions. Thus, behavior was altered during the initial drug exposure and the subjects responded to the change in drug state during subsequent test sessions. These results suggested that nicotine produced an effect which could best be described as a state dependent (StD) effect. Therefore, a series of studies were designed to investigate the specific stimulus qualities of nicotine.

II. BEHAVIORAL APPROACHES USED TO STUDY THE STIMULUS PROPERTIES OF NICOTINE

A. State Dependent Learning (StD) vs Discriminative Stimulus (DS) Paradigms

The stimulus properties of psychoactive drugs can be studied utilizing either StD or DS paradigms. According to the StD procedure, subjects are trained to perform a specific task under drug or non-drug conditions. During the testing phase of the procedure, the drug and non-drug groups are divided and half of each group is tested for retention under drug or non-drug conditions. Drugs which produce StD effects exhibit asymetric learning deficits across this 2 x 2 design when testing rats in the absence of the drug after they had been trained under the drug state. Thus, learning a specific task in this procedure appears to be contingent upon the drug being administered during training phases. Several behavioral tasks have been studied with this procedure including passive and active avoidance paradigms.

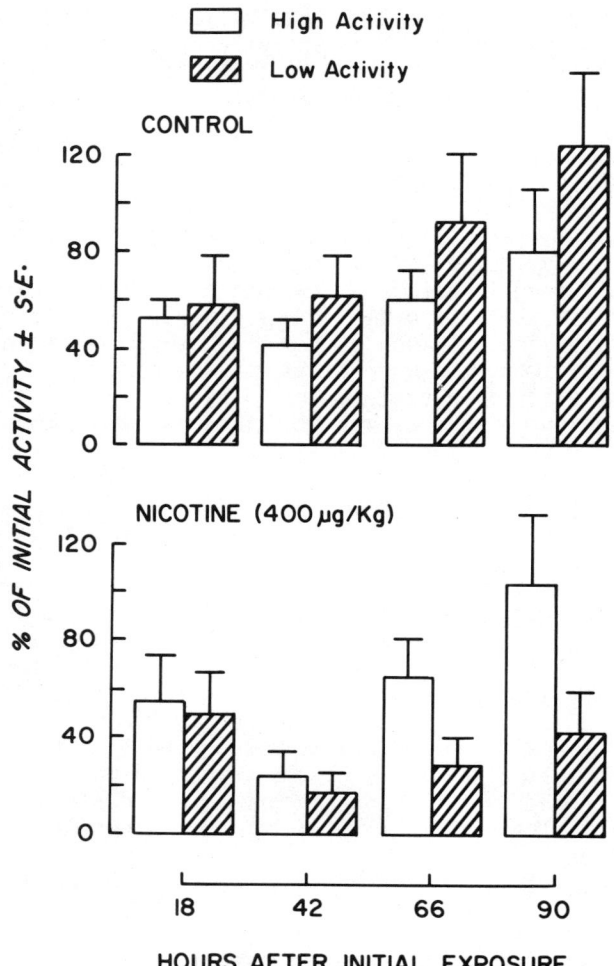

Figure 1. Effects on nicotine on rate of habituation in high and low activity rats. Rats of both activity groups (n=40) were administered either nicotine (400 μg/kg;sc) or saline and immediately placed in a square activity cage (Lafayette Instruments, Lafayette, Ind.) for 15 min. Animals were returned to the apparatus at 18 hour and then at 24 hour intervals for 15 min. and activity recorded. Data provided above represents the % change of initial activity during subsequent sessions. Nicotine did not alter behavior during the initial exposure.

Under the discriminative stimulus procedure, rats are trained to respond differentially under each drug state. Within this paradigm, the drug serves as a discriminative stimulus and is similar to a specific sensory discriminative stimulus. According to the DS procedures, the animals learn to obtain positive reinforcement (food or water) or avoid shock under specific drug states and are usually trained using a two-bar operant chamber or T-maze apparatus. Thus, the DS procedure allows the animal to identify the drug state.

Whether these two approaches constitute the same qualitative drug effect is debatable. Some authors insist that the difference is essentially quantitative with both DS and StD properties of psychoactive drugs being produced through similar mechanisms. Our experience has suggested that the DS paradigm is most sensitive for the specific investigation of the behavioral effects of nicotine. An advantage of the DS procedure is that learning to discriminate between drug states is contingent upon the subject becoming behaviorally tolerant to the specific drug. Thus, with this procedure one does not have to be concerned with the disruptive behavioral effects of the drug. These disruptive effects can be a source of confounding error in procedures which utilize a drug only once or twice as in the StD paradigms. In this situation the lack of tolerance may be observed to interfere with the performance of the response needed to demonstrate learning.

B. State Dependent Properties of Nicotine

Earlier experiments indicated that nicotine produced an apparent StD change in behavior (Fig. 1). Therefore, one of our first tasks was to decide upon a procedure with which to study the StD effects of nicotine. Across these studies, four procedures were utilized: (1) a positive reinforcement paradigm, (2) a passive avoidance paradigm, (3) a conditioned emotional response (CER) paradigm, and (4) unsignaled avoidance behavior. The overall approach in each of these procedures was to train rats on a given task under drug and non-drug conditions and then study retention under a reversed drug state. In the first procedure rats were exposed to a circular open field maze for 15 minutes, water-deprived for 48 hours, and again placed in the apparatus with access to water (water bottle was also present during the initial exposure). In this procedure, rats previously exposed to the apparatus will exhibit a faster latency to drink than rats not exposed to it. It was anticipated that exposed rats receiving nicotine would respond like the non-exposed saline-injected group, thus indicating a StD effect of the drug. The results of this experiment (Table 1) show that a very different effect was observed. Analysis of the data pooled across activity levels indicated no difference between the nicotine and saline treatments. If the data were separated into subgroups of activity level, however, nicotine was found to increase the time to drink in the high activity group and decrease this parameter in the low activity group. Thus, these results again suggest that nicotine produced a subtle behavioral change resulting from habituation-baseline behavior interactions rather than a StD effect.

Another StD procedure involved a CER paradigm (Table 2). In this procedure fear was conditioned in rats to 3 shocks paired with a white noise at 20 sec (random) intertrail intervals. The white noise (CS) preceeded a 1 ma shock (US) by 2 sec and terminated with

TABLE 1

Effects of Nicotine on Habituation Rate:
An Approach to Studying State Dependent Learning[a]

Activity Groups	Control n=20	Nicotine n=20	% Change
Pooled groups	2.41 ± 0.78	2.89 ± 0.79	+19%
High activity	1.19 ± 0.39	4.50 ± 0.09	+278% $p < 0.01$
Low activity	3.63 ± 1.39	1.23 ± 0.77	-66% $p < 0.001$

[a] Values represent time to begin drinking after rats were placed in an open field procedure exposed to 48 hrs. prior for 15 mins. under either the nicotine (400 µg/kg) or saline state.

the 2 sec duration shock. Three days later the rats were placed in a circular path activity cage (Woodward Industries, Herdon, Va.) for 3 min. and white noise was again presented at 20 sec intervals with activity levels being recorded at the termination of each session. As can be observed (Table 2), the activity levels of the saline-injected rats were reduced, indicating that the CS evoked a conditioned suppression response. Asymetric dissociation was not observed with either nicotine dosage (200 or 400 µg/kg) studied. According to the StD model, the nicotine-saline group should not have responded to the CER and their activity levels should not have been different from the non-shock controls. Instead at the 400 µg/kg dose of nicotine, the CER responses were potentiated in both the nicotine-nicotine groups. This effect was apparently produced during the training phase of the 2 x 2 design, since the saline-nicotine group showed no similar suppression of activity.

A further investigation of this phenomenon was made using a passive avoidance paradigm to study the effects of the same doses of nicotine within a 2 x 2 design. In this task rats were placed in a circular brightly illuminated open field maze with an opening to a dark cage (centrally located) which could be electrified. The animals were allowed exposure for a maximum time of 300 sec during both the training and testing phases of the study. The rats initially entered the dark cage with a mean latency of 11.7 sec. After entering, the subjects were given 10 1-sec shocks (1 ms) across a 1 min. exposure. At the 200 µg/kg dosage of nicotine an asymetrical dissociation was evident, but the decrease in latency to enter the shocked cage was also lowered in the nicotine-nicotine group.

The last investigation of StD phenomenon associated with nicotine involved a shuttle avoidance procedure using an unsignaled

TABLE 2

State Dependent Effects of Nicotine in Two Experimental Passive Avoidance Procedure[a]

Drug Regimen Training-Testing	CER Counts		Passive Avoidance Interquartile Range	
	200 µg/kg	400 µg/kg	200 µg/kg	400 µg/kg
Saline-Saline	112	---	271	---
Saline-Nicotine	137	102	279	269
Nicotine-Saline	115	25[b]	12[b]	281
Nicotine-Nicotine	128	29[b]	72	284

[a]Two procedures were studied, a Conditioned Emotional Response (C.E.R., n=12 for each value) and Passive Avoidance (P.A.) Procedure (n=15 for each value). Data collected during testing sessions activity of controls not receiving C.E.R.= 223 ± 21 during a 3-min. exposure in a circular path activity cage. Control entrance time in the P.S. procedure = 11.7 sec for rats under drug and non-drug states during training; values were reported as in the interquartile range (75% score - 25% score, Rank 11 - Rank 5) during test procedures.

[b]Significance $p < 0.05$; student "t" in C.E.R. procedure and rank sum test in P.A. procedure.

paradigm (Sigman Avoidance Procedure). In this study, nicotine (400 µg/kg, sc) facilitated learning by high-active rats and tended to reduce the learning ability of low-active rats. Again there was no evidence of a StD effect when either group of rats was shifted to the non-drug state. Thus, performance during training under the nicotine state and testing under the non-drug state did not show any differential effect.

These experiments, as with previous studies, illustrated consistent effects of nicotine on the variables associated with learning. Any StD activity of the drug, however, was confounded by other pharmacological effects which appeared related to motivation and memory mechanisms. Therefore, classic StD effects of the drug were not observed in any of the procedures. These investigations of StD effects of nicotine, however, may have generated data helpful in explaining why man finds the drug reinforcing. The most consistent finding from the animal studies is the modulating effect of nicotine on baseline activity rates. Although similar behavioral changes have not been reported in man, these modulating effects of the drug may be expressed as subtle changes in CNS neural activity. These studies also suggest that nicotine may enhance learning, but whether this effect occurs via changes in memory, motivation, or performance is not clear.

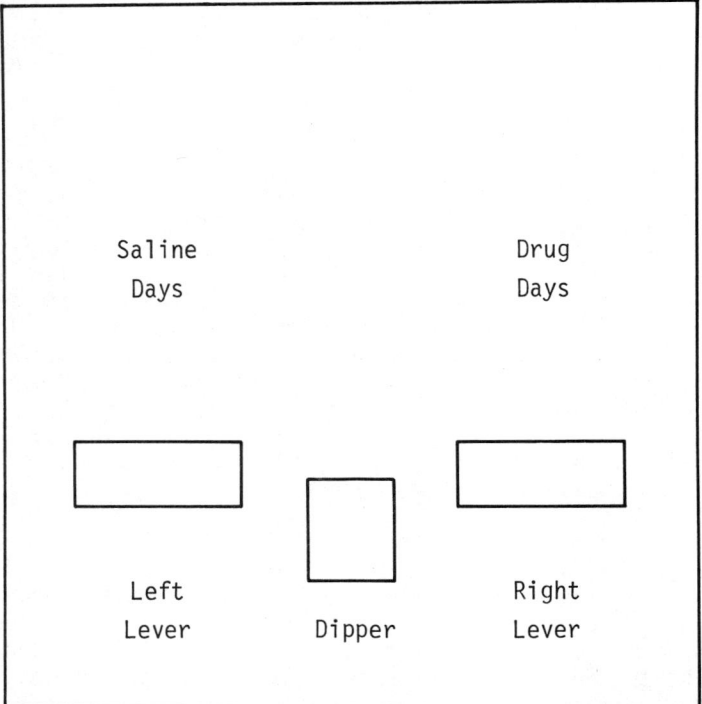

Figure 2. A representation of the drug discrimination training procedure. Rats were trained on one lever while under saline and the oppostie lever was reinforced while under the nicotine state. Lever side and drug administration was assigned randomly and counter-balanced to avoid preferences.

C. Nicotine as a Discriminative Stimulus (DS)

Concurrent with the above StD approaches, the ability of nicotine to act as a DS was extensively studied (Schechter and Rosecrans, 1971a-b). The procedures used in these investigations were the T-maze and the two-lever operant paradigms (Schechter and Rosecrans, 1971a; Hirschhorn and Rosecrans, 1974a). Early investigations used the T-maze procedure in both positively reinforced and escape tasks, while our later research has concentrated on the use of the two-lever operant procedure. There are several reasons for this change in experimental design, which are important to studying drugs as discriminative stimuli. The T-maze task was abandoned because (1) higher doses of the drug were needed to train rats, (2) the all or nothing nature of the data served to complicate dose-response and drug-generalization tests, and (3) strain differences interacted with the procedure, i.e. Sprague Dawley rats experienced great difficulty in learning the escape procedures. The usefulness of the T-maze paradigm appears to be limited to the identification and classification of the stimulus properties of a drug or groups of drugs. Most of these problems are circumvented through the use of the two-lever operant procedure. Using this paradigm, the rats are free to respond at any rate on either bar, and the data can be expressed in terms of % correct-bar responding. Overall, we have found the two-bar operant paradigm to be more specific and sensitive as a technique to study the DS effects of psychoactive drugs.

The two-bar operant procedure used involves training food-deprived rats to press both bars for liquid food reinforcement prior to the administration of any drug. Drug-training begins with two sessions under each drug state (nicotine or saline), with each bar being reinforced (CRF schedule) depending upon the drug administered (Fig.2). These daily drug-training sessions are initiated 10 min after the s.c. injection of nicotine or saline and are run on a 5 day/wk basis, according to a double alternation procedure and a specific schedule or partial reinforcement. In most of these studies the first 2.5 min of each session are not reinforced. These "extinction" sessions allow for the collection of learning data under the discriminative control of the drug removed from the biasing effect of reinforcement (Fig. 3).

Nicotine usually assumes stimulus control of operant behavior within 20 single sessions under each drug state. The effects of the duration of the training sessions were studied across 2 time periods (15 and 30 min) under two doses of nicotine (100 and 200 µg/kg). As can be observed (Table 3) the rats at both doses learned faster during the shorter training sessions. Apparently the 30 min session did not provide for faster learning because of either motivational (satiation or fatigue) factors or early (within the first 15 min) peak drug levels. The data collected during these studies was expressed at % correct responding on the nicotine-correct lever. Thus, rats who learn to discriminate nicotine should make at least 80% of their total responses on the nicotine-correct lever when under the nicotine state and less than 25% on the same lever after the injection of saline. The difference between these 2 values is the level of drug discriminability. Most of the research reported in this chapter was collected during the

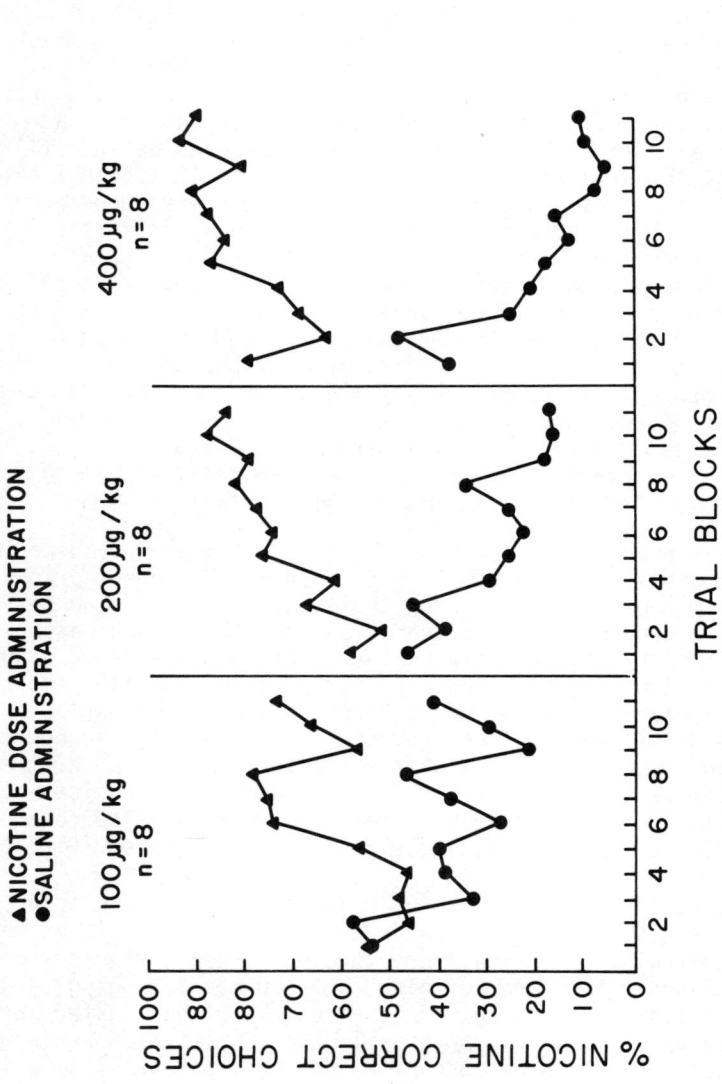

Figure 3. Nicotine discrimination learning curves at three dose levels under a VI-15 sec schedule of reinforcement. Each trial block represents two training sessions under one drug state which were presented via a double alternation sequence. Data was collected during 2.5 min extinction periods presented at the beginning of each training session.

2.5 min nonreinforced test sessions interspaced between two training blocks under the nicotine and saline states. It should be added that the training sessions were also preceeded by 2.5 min test sessions, preventing the subjects from detecting differences between testing and training sessions.

TABLE 3

Rates of Learning the Nicotine Stimulus[a]

Time (min.)	100 µg/kg	200 µg/kg
15	37.5	40.8
30	28.7	37.5
% change	+ 34%	+ 32%

[a]Data are presented as mean discriminability values (responses on the nicotine correct lever under nicotine minus responses on the nicotine correct lever under saline) of rats trained to discriminate between both drug states. Each value represents the mean of 6 rats and data was collected during sessions 3-15 of training; 12 exposures under each drug state.

This masking of the testing sessions is important if one is to obtain correct evaluations of dose-response and drug-generalization tests. The mechanism of action of nicotine was studied through the use of drug antagonists. These agents were administered prior to a specific nicotine training-dose % nicotine-correct responding was determined. A second strategy was to compare the stimulus effects of known and unknown compounds with nicotine as a means of evaluating the sensitivity and specificity of the nicotine stimulus. This evaluation was accomplished by injecting the nicotine-trained rats with the compound and measuring their % responding on the nicotine- and saline-correct bars. This same strategy has also proven useful in the evaluation of several nicotine-like compounds (cotinine and amphetamine).

III. SENSITIVITY AND SPECIFICITY OF THE STIMULUS

A. Dose-Response and Time-Duration Experiments

Several studies were designed to determine the sensitivity of the nicotine stimulus. The strength of the nicotine stimulus appeared proportional to the training dose across 20 exposures to the drug and saline states (Fig. 3). Over time, however, the rats exhibited fewer differences between the doses, and the % discriminability was equal across the doses of the drug, indicating similar stimulus strengths. A further evaluation of the sensitivity of the stimulus was tested during dose-generalization studies conducted during the monreinforced test session (Table 4). The sensitivity, as measured by the ED-50 dose, appeared proportional to the training dose, but was asymptotic above 200 µg/kg. Thus, the stimulus effects of 200 and 400 µg/kg were equipotent after the drug has assumed discriminative control of the operant behavior. Additional studies (Hirschhorn and Rosecrans, 1974) again indicate that differences in stimulus strength across doses of nicotine are more related to the training phase than to the sensitivity of the animals to the drug once the DS has been learned.

TABLE 4

Nicotine Dose Generalization Involving Different Schedules and Training Doses

Dose and Schedule [a]	(n)	ED-50 Dose µg/kg (95% C.L.)
VI-15; 100 µg/kg	(8)	26 (9-71)
VI-15; 200 µg/kg	(8)	79 (40-161)
VI-15; 400 µg/kg	(8)	86 (40-185)
FR-10; 400 µg/kg	(6)	98 (42-184)
Drl-10; 400 µg/kg	(6)	93 (40-215)

[a] Dose-response studies were conducted during non-reinforced test sessions. Doses were ½, ¼ and 1/8 of the training dose and ED-50's were calculated via the procedures of Litchfield and Wilcoxin (1949). An analysis of variance indicated that the VI-15; 100 µg/kg was significant from 400 µg/kg dose at $p < 0.025$. None of the other data presented were significant.

Because of the variable effect of nicotine on baseline rates of behavior, the stimulus properties of the drug were studied in rats trained under different schedules of reinforcement (Murphin, 1974). These studies indicate that few differences in discrimination existed across the training phase of the study, since the ED-50 doses did not differ across the schedules (Table 4). Thus, although the rates of responding differed across the schedules (Table 6), there was no significant differences in % discrimination. These schedules, therefore, appear equally sensitive to generalizations of stimulus control across various doses of the drug.

The time-duration parameters of the nicotine stimulus have also been investigated (Hirschhorn and Rosecrans, 1974a) using a VI-15 schedule of reinforcement (Fig.4). The stimulus effect following the administration of 400 µg/kg, s.c. was evident for at least 60 minutes and began to approach chance levels 80 minutes after the injection. Similar studies have also been conducted comparing the duration of the stimulus effect across various schedules of reinforcement (Murphin, 1974). No significant differences in the duration of the stimulus effects of nicotine were observed across DRL-10, FR-10, or VI-15 schedules. Thus, as indicated for the ED-50 data, the stimulus was equally sensitive in relation to the duration of effect.

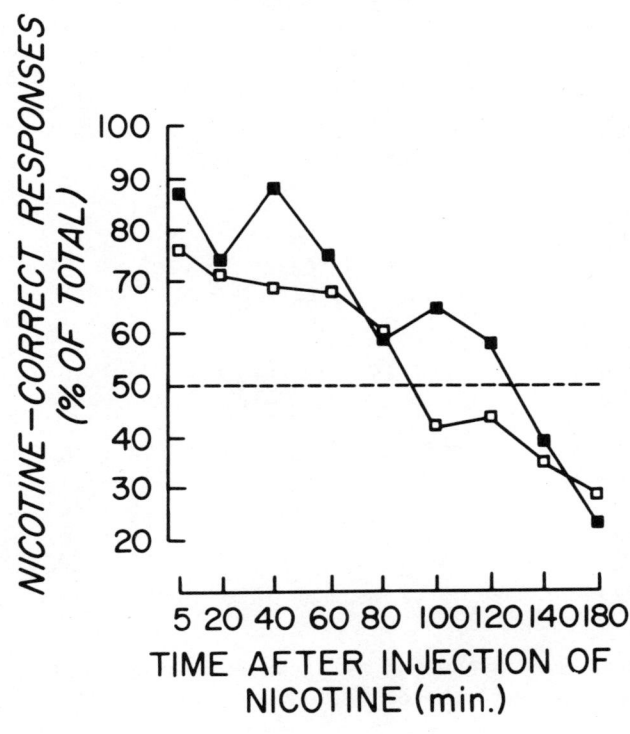

Figure 4. Time-duration generalization curves for rats trained to discriminate nicotine from saline states. Rats were administered a dose of nicotine and placed in the operant chamber at various times thereafter. Data was collected during 2.5 min non-reinforced test sessions between two training blocks of nicotine and saline; n=6 for each dose.

B. Specificity of the Nicotine Stimulus

Investigations of the specificity of the nicotine stimulus effect is extremely important if one is to use such a procedure as a model for studying drug mechanisms. Thus, several studies were initiated to determine to which compounds nicotine would generalize. Initial studies using the T-maze procedure found no generalization to muscarinic agonists, alkaloids (lobeline), or to any other drug tested (Schechter and Rosecrans, 1972a-d; 1973).

Assessment of the stimulus effect of d-amphetamine and its generalization to nicotine was initiated, since several investigators had reported some similarities between this drug and nicotine. Although initial studies indicated that the stimulus properties of these two drugs were perceived as different, another study was designed to investigate the generalization of nicotine to d-amphetamine under different schedules of reinforcement (Table 5).

TABLE 5

Generalization of Nicotine to Various Dose of d-Amphetamine[a]

Dose of d-Amphetamine µg/kg	VI-15 n=8	FR-10 n=6	DrI-10 n=6
0	11 + 3	11 + 5.6	24 + 10
60	14 + 7	6 + 4	17 + 11
120	30 + 12	21 + 12	26 + 24
240	34 + 10	7 + 6	55 + 12
480	44 + 13	18 + 11	20 + 20
720	54 + 16	33 + 33	46 + 21

[a] Values were presented as % correct responses on the nicotine lever; Nicotine = 400 µg/kg

Significant generalization of d-amphetamine to nicotine did not occur under any condition. These generalizations were generally inconsistent except within the VI-15 schedule a nonsignificant trend of increased % nicotine-correct responding with higher doses of d-amphetamine was observed. Thus, these subjects (VI-15) responded to d-amphetamine as being different from both saline and nicotine. Therefore, we inferred that the drug produced a qualitatively different effect than that produced by nicotine. Another important aspect of this study concerned the effects of d-amphetamine and nicotine on response rates (Table 6). While neither drug biased response rates when the rats were trained under the VI-15 schedule, similar increases of response rates were observed under both DRL and FR schedules following the injection of d-amphetamine. It is interesting to note that although this drug increased response rates, the % discrimination was not favored by this increase (Table 5). Furthermore, this relationship indicates the independent nature of both of these behavioral components. As observed in Tables 5 and 6, rates of responding and % discrimination reflect two different aspects of behavior, bearing little positive relationship to each other.

TABLE 6

Mean Response Rates Under Various Drug States:
Various Schedules of Reinforcement[a]

Drug State	Drl-10 n=4	VI-15 n=6	FR-10 n=6
Saline	8.5	27.0	40.0
Nicotine	8.6	27.8	61.2 (+ 53%)
d-Amphetamine	21.7 (+ 152%)	26.0	103.0 (+ 157%)

[a] Data are presented as mean response rates 1 min. on both levers under each drug state during 2.5 min. extinction or test sessions. Values represent the mean of six d-amphetamine (60-720-μg/kg, i.p.) and an equal number of saline and nicotine exposures. (400 μg/kg).

The data provided by this series of studies is important in that it firmly establishes the validity of the procedures we are using. The discriminative stimulus paradigm meets all the parmacological requirements to establish the technique as a profitable way of studying the mechanism of action of nicotine.

IV. CENTRAL NATURE OF THE NICOTINE STIMULUS

A. Peripheral vs Central Mechanisms

An important aspect of the nicotine stimulus effect concerns the possibility that the stimulus may be mediated by peripheral rather than central mechanisms. As previously stated, nicotine has been observed to have various effects on the peripheral autonomic nervous system. Included among these peripheral changes are increased blood pressure, changes in heart rate, and the release of epinephrine (E) and NE from the adrenal medulla. In addition, solutions of the drug are basis in pH and their injection could produce pain or other detectable sensory changes. We have attempted to answer this question through the use of several different approaches, but as yet cannot entirely eliminate the possibility of peripheral mediation of the nicotine cue. The first approach focused on the use of peripherally-acting vs centrally-acting nicotine antagonists. Thus, pretreatments with the centrally-active nicotinic antagonist, mecamylamine, was observed to effectively block the nicotine cue in the T-maze, while pretreatments with a nicotinic antagonist unable to pass the blood-brain barrier, hexamethonium, had no effect (Schechter and Rosecrans, 1971a). Another approach studied generalization to nicotine of the stimulus effects of a quarternary nicotine compound synthesized by Dr. H. McKennis, Jr. and colleagues (Schechter and Rosecrans, 1972). No evidence of generalization was found when this peripherally-acting nicotine compound was tested in nicotine-trained rats. Therefore, both of these approaches have generated data suggesting that the nicotine stimulus effect is mediated by central rather than peripheral mechanisms.

B. Nicotine Levels vs the Stimulus Effect

Another strategy used to investigate the central nature of the nicotine stimulus compared brain area nicotine levels with the drug's behavioral effect (Hirschhorn and Rosecrans, 1972; Schechter and Jellinek, 1975). Both groups of workers have provided ample evidence that before nicotine can act as a DS it must achieve a specific drug level in the brain.

While these data provide interesting information, these studies were conducted using acute nicotine dosages. Rosecrans (1972) has observed, however, that peak brain nicotine levels can shift depending upon whether 1 or 5 doses of the drug are administered. Therefore, an additional study was designed in which rats were injected with at least 80 nicotine and saline doses according to the schedule occurring in the behavioral DS paradigms (Fig.5). Three doses (200, 300 and 400 µg/kg) of nicotine were studied and the rats were sacrificed at 5 minutes intervals up to 30 minutes to determine the nicotine levels.

This period of time was chosen because most of our behavioral research has involved 15-30 minute training sessions. Dose-response relationships were evident across the 4 brain areas studied (cerebral cortex, limbic forebrain, diencephalon, and brainstem), and were the strongest in the cerebral cortex. Although these results correlated well with other studies, the peak drug levels were observed at different times, within different brain areas across different doses of the drug, suggesting many alternatives in the attempt to correlate brain area with drug effect. At this point we can state that nicotine must enter the brain to produce a stimulus effect. However, from the brain area nicotine distribution studies thus far conducted, we cannot be certain which brain area is specifically involved in the mediation of the stimulus effect.

C. Generalization to Intraventricular Doses of Nicotine

A third strategy in studying the central effect of nicotine is to measure the stimulus effects of the drug when it is injected directly into the brain. Schechter (1973) designed a series of studies indicating generalization of the stimulus effects from peripheral (400 µg/kg) to central (644 ng) administration of nicotine. He was also able to demonstrate generalization of central to peripheral administration of the drug using doses (644 ng) equivalent to those measured centrally after a peripheral injection.

As a means of further analyzing these findings, a series of studies were designed in which dose-response generalization from the s.c. to the intraventricular (ivt) routes of administration were compared (Fig. 6 and 7). Dose-response generalizations were apparent

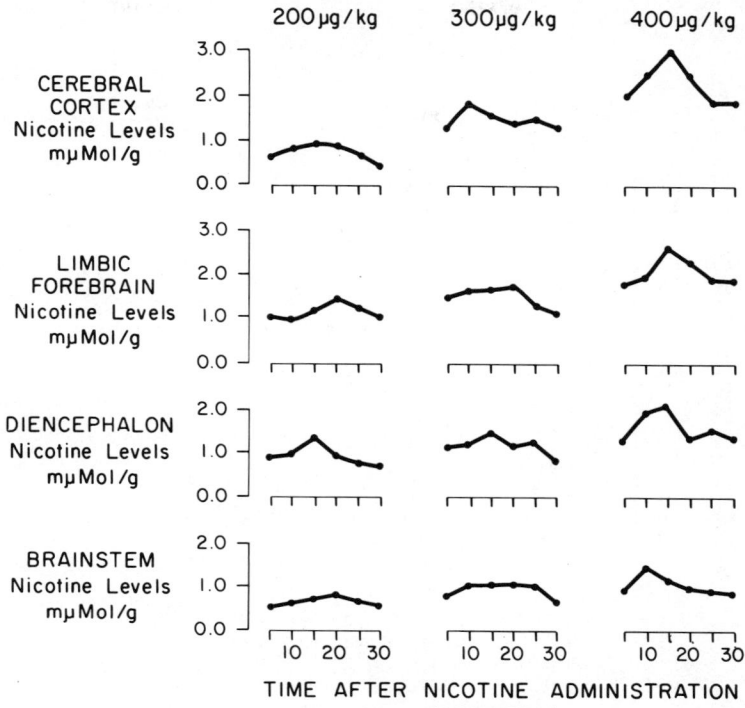

Figure 5. Brain area nicotine levels following various chronic dose of nicotine. Ninety male rats were given 80 nicotine and saline doses each on alternate days, 5 days/week. On the 80th day a tracer amount of (C^{14}) nicotine was added to drug solutions and animals sacrificed 5 min intervals up to 30 min (n=5 at each) after specific nicotine doses. Brain areas were frozen and nicotine levels measured as described previously (Rosecrans, 1972).

under all training conditions except in rats trained under the DRL-10 schedule. Generalization following the ivt injection of nicotine was rather complete, especially in rats trained at 400 μg/kg s.c. under the FR-10 and VI-15 schedules of reinforcement. Calculation of the generalization ED-50 doses (Table 7 revealed that in this study much higher ivt doses (9-20 μg) were required for generalization of the stimulation control than in the report by Schechter (0.6 μg). To further amplify this difference, calculation of the ED-50 on a per kg basis (Table 7) revealed that the total ivt dose was equal to that given peripherally (Table 4). This finding does not appear to be unusual for nicotine as Dr. M. Aceto (MCV, personal communication) has indicated that mice require similar doses of nicotine to produce convulsions whether the central or peripheral route of administration is used. At this point we have no explanation for these contradictory findings, except that Schechter used an escape paradigm while we used an appetite operant procedure. We have also attempted to train rats

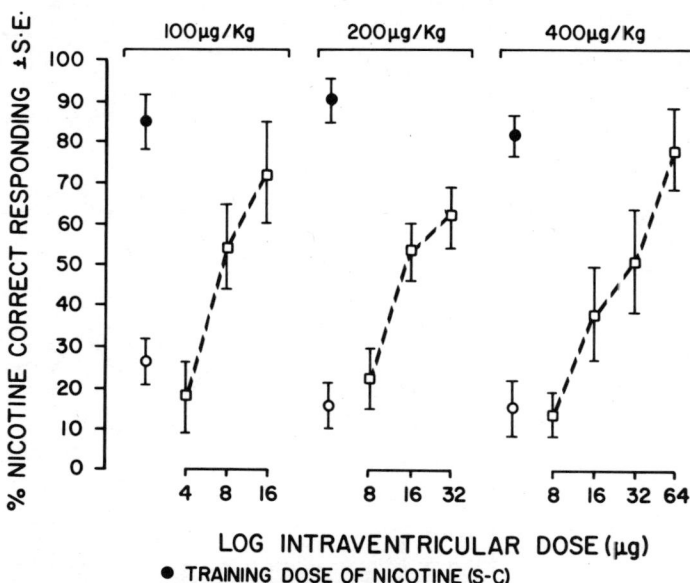

Figure 6. Stimulus generalization of nicotine from peripheral (sc) to control (iv) administration. The subjects employed in this study were the same as those in Figure 3.

to discriminate the stimulus effects of nicotine from saline using the ivt route of administration (Fig.8). These rats were unable to discriminate the drug states even at doses (16-32 μg) that previously produced good discrimination via the ivt route in the generalization studies (Figs. 6 and 7). At this point we have formulated the hypothesis that nicotine may be excreted from the ventricle very rapidly and then taken up into the brain via the usual peripheral routes. This hypothesis could explain why the peripheral and ivt doses are equivalent in the generalization studies, but several alternative explanations are also tenable.

D. Central Effects of Nicotine Metabolites

An alternative explanation of the above conflicting data is that nicotine is acting through an active metabolite formed at a peripheral site, such as the liver. To test this hypothesis, one of the more important metabolites of nicotine, cotinine (prepared by Dr. H. McKennis Jr., MCV), was administered through both the s.c. and ivt routes to nicotine-trained rats (Table 8). No generalization of cotinine to nicotine (400 μg/kg) was observed across two schedules of reinforcement (VI-15 and FR-10) even when 8 times the nicotine-training dose was

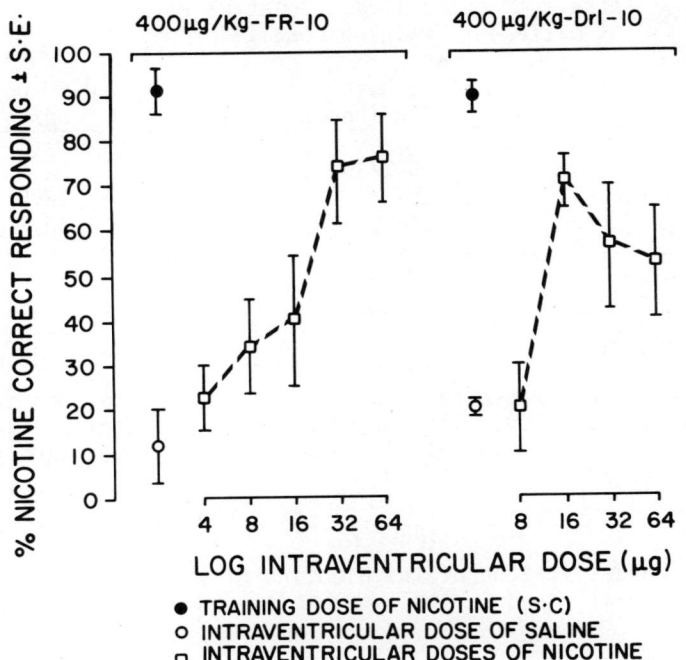

Figure 7. Stimulus generalization of nicotine from peripheral (sc) to control (iv) administration. Rats were trained to discriminate nicotine (400 µg/kg) from saline using Drl-10 and FR-10 schedules (n=6 for each).

given peripherally. When the two drugs were given via the ivt route, however, 16 µg of cotinine generalized to an equal amount of nicotine. This generalization occurred only in rats trained at 100 µg/kg, being much less potent when tested in those trained at 200 µg/kg of nicotine. These data suggest that nicotine is not producing its stimulus effects through metabolism to cotinine. The cotinine that does get into the brain, however, appears to elicit stimulus effects very similar to those of nicotine. The results of this study also indicate that different training doses may not just reflect different sensitivities to the same drug. The rats trained at 200 µg/kg of nicotine responded to cotinine less like nicotine than did the rats trained at 100 µg/kg, suggesting that these training doses were also qualitiatively different. It should be added that cotinine is the only metabolite of nicotine that we have studied. Thus, at this point much more research needs to be done to elucidate the differences in discrimination following central and peripheral administration of nicotine and its metabolites.

TABLE 7

Generalization of S.C. Administered Nicotine to Intraventricular (I.V.) Doses Under Different Training Conditions

Dose and Schedule[a]	ED-50 Dose (95% µg Confidence Limits)	ED-50 Dose µg/kg
VI-15; 100 µg/kg	9 (5-17)	22.5
VI-15; 200 µg/kg	13 (5-38)	32.5
VI-15; 400 µg/kg	20 (40-185)	50.0
FR-10; 400 µg/kg	14 (6-35)	35.0
Drl-10; 400 µg/kg	----	----

[a] Rats trained to discriminate under various dose and/or schedule were implanted with i.v. (left or right lateral ventricle) and administered various doses of nicotine. These animals were the same as presented in Table 2.

TABLE 8

Generalization of the Nicotine Stimulus to Peripherally and Centrally Administered Cotinine[a]

Drug and Dose	Peripheral Administration		Drug and Dose	Central Administration	
	VI-15 400 µg/kg	FR-10 400 µg/kg		VI-15 100 µg/kg	VI-15 200 µg/kg
Nicotine Training	84 ± 7	94 ± 4	Nicotine 16 µg	72 ± 8	
			32 µg		64 ± 11
Cotinine mg/kg			Cotinine µg		
0.40	-----	9 ± 4	8	34 ± 16	25 ± 10
0.50	19 ± 9	15 ± 4	16	74 ± 8	47 ± 15
1.60	23 ± 13	21 ± 2	32	-----	39 ± 14
3.20	36 ± 12	23 ± 10	64	31 ± 20	18 ± 15

[a] Values were presented as percent correct responses on the nicotine correct lever.

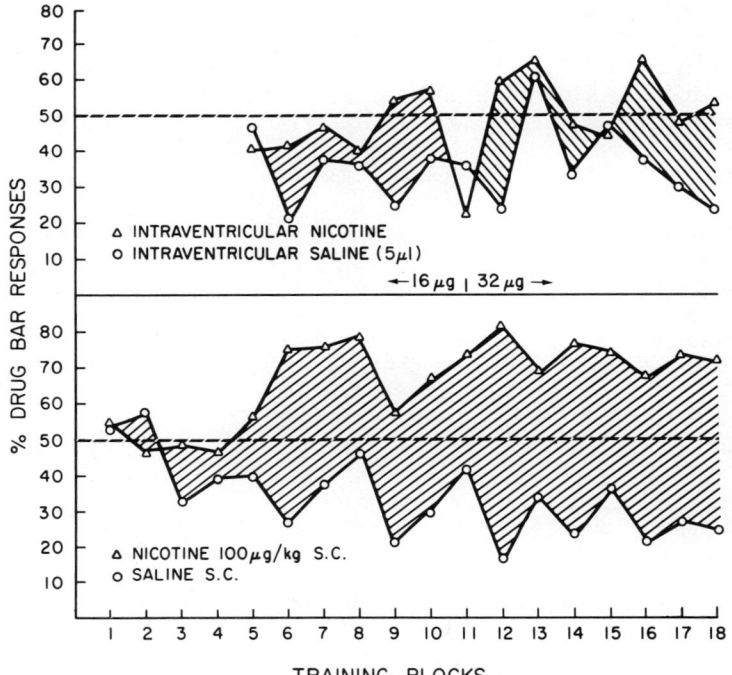

Figure 8. An attempt to train rats to discriminate nicotine vs. saline via either central or peripheral routes of administration (n=12 for each study). Procedures for each study were similar in terms of schedule (VI-15) and drug presentation (double alternation). Shaded areas reflect discriminability. Rats trained to discriminate nicotine vs. saline centrally were administered doses in 5 μl volumes via permanent cannulas.

V. CENTRAL CHOLINERGIC MECHANISMS

A. Drug Antagonism Studies

The general approach to studying cholinergic mechanisms of action was similar to that reported by Domino (1967). In these studies a series of N- and M-cholinergic antagonists were used as pretreatments to analyze the stimulus properties of nicotine (Hirschhorn and Rosecrans, 1974). The drugs were generally administered 10-30 minutes prior to a training dose of nicotine and % discrimination was determined during specific test sessions. Mecamylamine (N-cholinergic antagonist) was the only drug observed to completely antagonize the nicotine stimulus (Table 9). As the dose of this antagonist was increased, % correct responses on the nicotine-correct lever after the injection of 200 or 400 μg/kg of nicotine declined to saline response levels, indicating a complete antagonism of the nicotine stimulus. This antagonism also appeared to be competitive in nature, since the ED-50 (95% C.L.) doses indicated that a 331 (105-1039) μg/kg dose of mecamylamine antagonized the stimulus effects of

200 μg/kg of nicotine, while 835 (239-2913) μg/kg was required for similar antagonism of the 400 μg/kg dose of nicotine (Hirschhorn and Rosecrans, 1974a). This antagonism is reversible and also occurs within the brain, since the peripherally-acting N-cholinergic antagonist, hexamethonium, was also without effect. The M-cholinergic

TABLE 9

Mechanism of the Stimulus: Drug Antagonism Studies

Drug Antagonist	Receptor Blocked	Result vs Nicotine
Mecamylamine (s.c.) 1 mg/kg; 30 min. prior	N-cholinergic central acting	complete antagonism
Hexamethonium (s.c.) 1 mg/kg; 10 min. prior	N-cholinergic peripheral acting	no effect
Atropine (s.c.) 0.5-2.0 mg/kg; 30 min. prior	M-cholinergic central acting	no effect
Dibenamine (i.p.) 10-20 mg/kg; 30 min.	α-adrenergic	no effect
Propranolol (i.p.) 1-4 mg/kg	β-adrenergic	no effect
α-Methyl-paratyrosine (i.p.) 30-200 mg/kg; 2 hr. prior	catecholamine synthesis I	some blockade
p-Chlorophenylalanine (p.o.) 300 mg/kg; 72 hr. prior	5-hydroxytryptamine synthesis	no effect

antagonist, atropine, was also without effect against the nicotine stimulus, suggesting the existence of a separate N-cholinergic receptor. The possible relationships of the nicotine stimulus to NE and 5-HT systems were also investigated through the use of the appropriate antagonists and provided little support for the indirect involvement of these systems. There was a blockade by the NE synthesis inhibitor, alpha-methyl-paratyrosine (AMPT), but this effect may have been caused by a generalized decrease of arousal levels (Schechter and Rosecrans, 1972c). Thus unlike the peripheral ANS, the DS properties of nicotine appear singular and suggest the stimulation of a specific cholinergic receptor separate from the amine systems.

B. Muscarinic vs Nicotine DS Effects

While the above discussion is very suggestive of a specific central effect of the nicotine stimulus, other questions should be answered before we can adequately understand the basic cholinergic mechanisms of the effect. In addressing these questions, 3 studies were designed to investigate the DS properties of the M-cholinergic agonist arecoline. In the first study, arecoline was observed to assume DS control of operant behavior. The DS properties of arecoline were effectively blocked by pretreatments with the M-cholinergic antagonist, atropine, while the quarternary compound, methyl atropine (which does not readily cross the blood brain barrier, Rosecrans et al. 1968), was ineffective. These results indicate that stimulus control could be exerted via M-cholinergic stimulation and emphasize the central nature of the effect. Additional studies further indicated that mecamylamine was not able to antagonize the stimulus effects of arecoline (Schechter and Rosecrans, 1971b). Finally, Schechter and Rosecrans (1972c) were also able to train rats to discriminate the difference in stimulus effects of the M-and N-cholinergic agonists, arecoline and nicotine. Thus, there appears to be two independent central cholinergic receptor systems which exert stimulus control over behavior when appropriately stimulated. Our next task is to cetermine the site of these receptors within the CNS.

VI. INVOLVEMENT OF 5-HT SYSTEMS

A. Antagonism and Stimulation Studies

As indicated earlier in this chapter, a hypothesis concerning the effect of nicotine on 5-HT systems was initially proposed in order to account for its behavioral pharmacology. While not completely inclusive, two studies investigating the interactions of this amine system with the nicotine stimulus effect were designed. In the first study (Schechter and Rosecrans, 1972c), the stimulus properties of nicotine were evaluated in rats that had been depleted of 5-HT by pretreatments with the synthesis inhibitor, para-cholorophenylalamine (PCPA). As indicated in Table 9, these treatments did not alter the nicotine stimulus. The second strategy employed electrical stimulation of 5-HT systems within the midbrain raphe nuclei (MRN) as a DS (Hirschhorn, Hayes and Rosecrans, 1975). In this study rats readily learned to discriminate between the stimulated and nonstimulated conditions and generalized the electrically-induced DS to stimuli produced by LSD. When nicotine was administered to the rats trained to discriminate MRN stimulation, no generalization to the stimulus effects of the drug was observed, at doses ranging from 50 - 200 µg/kg. Therefore, the DS effects of nicotine do not appear to depend upon interactions with the 5-HT system.

VII. INVOLVEMENT OF CATECHOLAMINE SYSTEMS

A. An Overview of the Problem

Investigations of the interaction of the nicotine stimulus with catecholamine neuronal systems have yielded conflicting results. Thus Schechter and Rosecrans (1972c) observed that pretreatment of rats with the reversible inhibitor of catecholamine synthesis, AMPT, effectively obviated the discriminative stimulus effect of nicotine in a T-maze appetitive/adversive paradigm. Hirschhorn and Rosecrans (1974a), however, reported that pretreatments with AMPT had no effect upon nicotine controlled discrimination in the two-bar operant procedure.

The major difference in these two paradigms as used for the assessment of stimulus effects is that incorrect responses were punished in the T-maze and the data is based on one trial/day, while the two-bar operant task involved continuous responding for food reinforcement.

Similar disparities have also been observed with the stimulus effects of morphine and it's antagonism by PCPA, an inhibitor of serotonin biosynthesis. Again in these studies, pretreatment with PCPA blocked discriminative control by morphine in the T-maze procedure, while having no effect when the stimulus effects were assessed by the two-bar operant task (Rosecrans et al., 1973; Hirschhorn and Rosecrans, 1974b). Therefore, these data suggest that the interaction of nicotine stimulus effects with catecholamine systems may be related to the experimental paradigm used to assess these stimulus effects. Thus, the probability of a biochemical antagonism of a drug's stimulus effects appears greater if an adversive task is used in which correct responses are all or none (T-maze), than if the stimulus effects are assessed within an appetitive procedure based on continuous responding (two-bar operant).

B. An Approach to Studying DA and NE

To further evaluate the interaction between catecholamine systems with nicotine's stimulus properties a series of studies were conducted in which nicotine was studied in rats permanently depleted of dopamine (DA) or norepinephrine (NE). Nicotine (400 µg/kg) was studied using an appetitive VI-15 schedule or reinforcement. Amines were depleted in rats 14 days of age or younger via the technique of (Breese, 1975). The procedure was accomplished as follows: (1) norepinephrine was selectively depleted by the injection of 25 µg of 6-hydroxydopamine (6-OHDA) contained in 25 µl of behicle (5% ascorbic acid in normal saline) into the cisterna magna of one group of rats at both 1 and 7 days of age, (2) selective depletion of brain dopamine (DA) was accomplished in another group of subjects by similar injections of 150 µg of 6-OHDA at 14 days of age 30 min. after pretreatment with 30 mg/kg of desmethylimipramine (i.p.). Biochemical estimations in analagous groups of rats at 10 months of age indicate brain-NE to be lowered by 50% in NE groups and brain-DA to be lowered by 70% in DA group. A third group of six control rats was injected with the vehicle (25 µl) at 7 days of age. Two hours after the depletion procedures, all rats were returned to their mothers. The subjects were weaned at 28 days of age and individually housed on ad lib food and water until they were 90 days old. At 90 days of age six rats from each group (NE, DA, and control) were food-deprived to 80% of their body weight and trained to press both levers of an operant chamber for sweetened milk and then trained to discriminate between nicotine (400 µg/kg) and saline.

C. Sensitivity of the Nicotine Stimulus in Rats Depleted of Brain DA or NE

Rats in each of the three groups learned to discriminate the stimulus effects of nicotine easily within 30 sessions under each drug state (Table 10). Although there were no significant differences between groups, the % discriminability in the DA group tended to be lowest, while in the NE group it was the highest. It should be noted that in the NE group responding on the nicotine correct lever when under the non-drug state was lower than in other groups, while responding under the drug was equal to the control group.

TABLE 10

Nicotine Correct Bar Responding in
Dopamine (DA↓) and Norepinephrine Depleted Rats

Experimental Group	Amine Level[a] DA/NE S.E.	Nicotine % ± S.E.	Saline % ± S.E.
Control	3.76 ± 0.25 (15)	97 ± 3 (6)	24 ± 7
NE↓	5.38 ± 0.38 (15) + 43%	96 ± 3 (5)	11 ± 9
DA↓	1.72 ± 0.28 (15) − 54%	83 ± 7 (6)	24 ± 6

[a] The DA/NE value was calculated in 45 rats prepared in the same manner as in the behavioral study.

[b] Values represent % correct bar responding on the nicotine lever under each drug state. Each received 30 training under each drug state and the data represents the group average of six extention sessions ± S.E.

Results of the nicotine dose-generalization studies indicate that the ED-50 agonist dose was increased in both depleted groups. Furthermore, increases appeared greated in the NE group (Table 11), with NE depletion increasing the ED-50 dose by more than 60%. The dose of mecamylamine required to effectively block the stimulus effects of nicotine in half of the subjects (AD-50) was decreased in both of the catecholamine-depleted groups. This decrease was especially evident in DA rats in which the AD-50 dose was lowered by 40%. It should be emphasized that none of these data are statistically significant. They are however, suggestive.

The next strategy in these investigations was to inject nicotine directly into a highly cholinergic brain structure. To permit the injections, 24 ga cannulae were bilaterally implanted into the hippocampus of NE, DA, and control rats. Bilateral administration of nicotine (0.5 µg/µl saline) directly into the hippocampus in both NE and control rats appeared to elicit effective stimulus effects of the drug. Although discriminability was lower than when the drug was given peripherally, these animals did appear to discriminate between the stimulus effects of nicotine and saline following central administration (Table 12). Effective stimulus control of responding was

TABLE 11

Dose Transfer and Mecamylamine
Antagonism Studies in Nicotine Trained Rats

Experimental Group	(n)	Nicotine ED-50 μg/kg	Mecamylamine[a] AD-50 μg/kg
Control	(6)	85 (51-139)	620 (240-1320)
DA↓	(5)	97 (44-211)	390 (160-930)
NE↓	(6)	142 (95-210)	492 (260-920)

[a] Values presented represent either agonist or antagonist ED-50 data (95% Confidence Limits) obtained via the Litchfield and Wilcoxon procedure (1948). These data were also subjected to an analysis of variance; none of the data was significant beyond < 0.1.

never evident in DA rats following intrahippocampal injections of nicotine. In this group nicotine correct lever responding was lower following nicotine (5%) than when given saline (22%). Thus, although these DA subjects were capable of discriminating nicotine from saline, no evidence of this behavior could be elicited from hippocampal application of the drug.

If nicotine does produce some of its effects via the DA system then l-amphetamine rather than d-amphetamine might be recognized, more similar in terms of stimulus properties (Rosecrans et al., 1976). Such an experiment was conducted in rats trained to discriminate 200 μg/kg nicotine on a VI-15 schedule (Table 13). In contrast to what was expected nicotine-trained rats responded more on the nicotine-correct lever when under the d- rather than when under the l-amphetamine state. While not supporting our hypothesis the data again supports previous findings (Table 5) which indicate that the VI-15 schedule was more sensitive than other schedules in relation to detecting nonspecific central drug effects. The fact that doses over 400 μg/kg of d- or l-amphetamine suppressed response rates also suggests that these nicotine-trained rats were not cross tolerant to these stimulants.

D. Development of a Hypothesis

The previous study was designed to evaluate the effects of depletion of NE and DA upon the discriminative stimulus effects of nicotine. Although the data were not statistically significant, some suggestive trends did emerge from their interpretation.

It appears that the nicotine stimulus effects are not as potent in catecholamine-depleted rats. The NE group presents an interesting paradox, in that they appeared to be more sensitive to nicotine in

TABLE 12

Discriminability of Nicotine from Saline in Catecholamine Depleted Rats: Peripheral and Hippocampal Injections

Experimental Group	Peripheral Injection[a] 400 µg/kg	Hippocampal Injection[a] 1 µg/area
Control (N=5)	79% (5)[b]	33% (10)[b]
NE↓ (n=4)	65% (5)	23% (6)
DA↓ (n=4)	58% (5)	0% (7)

[a] Discriminability values = % nicotine correct responses after nicotine substracted by % nicotine correct responding after saline.

[b] Values in parenthesis represent replications in these rats; replication of each drug state.

TABLE 13

Generalization of Nicotine to d- and l-Amphetamine: VI-15 Schedules[a]

Dose	d-Amphetamine n=8	l-Amphetamine n=12
0	20.0 ± 4.1	19.9 ± 8.8
120	42.1 ± 13.4	20.6 ± 9.3
240	39.5 ± 12.1	22.3 ± 9.7
480	60.5 ± 9.7	26.1 ± 13.9

[a] Two separate groups of rats trained to discriminate nicotine at the 200 µg/kg dose were given various d- and l-amphetamine doses. Data was collected % correct responses on the nicotine lever.

terms of % discrimination (Table 10) and yet required a higher ED-50 dose (Table 11) of the drug. Examination of Table 11 reveals that the increase in % discrimination was due primarily to a decrease in saline-incorrect responding under the nicotine state. These results suggest that NE depletion may have made the rats more sensitive to the specific stimulus effects of nicotine (% D), while also producing decreased sensitivity to extraneous, arousal-type effects of the drug. Previous research (Rosecrans, 1970a) indicates that the NE system is excitatory and may function to maintain higher arousal levels. It is suggested that NE animals might be less affected by extraneous or nonspecific stimuli because of a lowered arousal level, and thus be better able to detect the nicotine stimulus. If central nicotinic-cholinergic-adrenergic interactions, similar to those of the peripheral autonomic nervous system, exist, elimination of NE from the system may produce the effects reported in this study. The observation that intrahippocampal injections of nicotine elicited appropriate stimulus effects in NE, however, suggests that NE is not essential for the perception of the nicotine stimulus effects.

Depletion of DA seems to have more dramatically affected perception of the nicotine stimulus. The DA group showed the worst performance in discrimination (Table 10), required less mecamylamine to block the stimulus effects (Table 11), and the ED-50 dose of nicotine was slightly increased (Table 11). More importantly, no evidence of nicotine stimulus control of operant responding was observed following intrahippocampal application of nicotine in the DA group (Table 12). The observation, however, that DA rats did learn to discriminate nicotine from saline suggests that the hippocampus is not the only site important to the perception of the nicotine stimulus. This finding also suggests that the nicotinic-cholinergic input or output of the hippocampus may depend upon the integrity of a DA system. Future research is being directed toward an investigation of whether this relationship is dependent upon a direct stimulation of DA neurons, release of DA, or a nicotinic-cholinergic interaction with DA systems.

VIII. SUMMARY AND CONCLUSIONS

A. Effects of Nicotine on Behavior

We have observed nicotine to produce very subtle but powerful effects on behavior. In addition we have also obtained some insight as to why nicotine could be reinforcing in man. The homeostatic effect of nicotine on behavior suggests how the drug could be used. If too excited, the drug could lower arousal while if sedated a stimulatory effect could ensue. In a sense it appears to be the perfect tranquilizer. Nicotine produces powerful state change in that what is learned is retained more than in the control state. Whether this is related to a memory or sensory mechanism is not understood at this time. This effect is also translatable in terms of its stimulus properties. Thus, a compound with such a powerful state-change capacity would be expected to evoke proportionately powerful discriminative stimulus effects. Integrating the data from the animal studies suggests several explanations of why man uses this reinforcing drug. What needs to be done now is to extend some of these studies to man.

B. Site and Mechanism of Nicotine's Behavioral Effects

The data provided from our research provides substantial evidence showing that nicotine is working upon very specific receptors within the brain. These receptors appear to be cholinergic in nature, but appear different from muscarinic (M-cholinergic) receptors. These studies have possibly suggested the hipoocampus as one specific site. This area does not appear to be the only brain-sensitive site, however, since there appears to be a dopaminergic link.

C. The Future

The DS approach provides us with a unique tool with which to study nicotine. It's effectiveness is dependent upon the ability of an animal to recognize drug vs. non-drug states, which appears contingent upon the stimulation of specific pharmacological receptors. We need not concern ourselves with other behavioral effects because of the specificity of this dependent variable. We can now characterize nicotine's stimulus effects in very exact terms much like we can do in isolated intestine studies. Thus, the time is right to go directly into the brain to ask where nicotine acting via the direct application of drug or by attempting to mimic the stimulus by electrical stimulation. We have the tools to create new animal strains in which to mainipulate those other non-cholinergic elements which can also influence nicotine's effects. Finally, we must also attempt to parallel these studies with very precise ones in humans. Therefore, we know the direction, we must only follow the signs. Unfortunately, in todays world of drug abuse problems, few find the time to explore how nicotine is working, a drug which is used by millions of humans throughout the world each day.

IX. REFERENCES

Bovet, D., Bovet-Nitti, F. and Oliverio, A.: Action of nicotine on spontaneous and acquired behavior in rats and mice. N.Y. Acad. Sci. 142:216-244, 1967.

Breese, G.R.: Chemical and immunochemical lesions by specific neurotoxic substances and antisera: Handbook of Psychopharmacology, ed by: L.L. Iverson, S.D. Iverson and S.H. Snyder, 1:137-189, 1975.

Domino, E.F.: Electroencephalographic and behavioral arousal effects of small doses of nicotine: A neuropsychological study. N.Y. Acad. Sci. 142:216-244, 1967.

Hirschhorn, I.D. and Rosecrans, J.A.: Studies on the time course and the effect of cholinergic and adrenergic receptor blockers on the stimulus effect of nicotine. Psychopharmacology 40:109-120, 1974a.

Hirschhorn, I.D. and Rosecrans, J.A.: A comparison of the stimulus effects of morphine and lysergic acid diethylamide (LSD). Pharmacol. Biochem. Behav. 2:361-366, 1974b.

Hirschhorn, I.D., Hayes, R.L., and Rosecrans, J.A.: Discriminative control of behavior by electrical stimulation of the dorsal raphe nucleus: Generalization to lysergic acid diethylamide (LSD). Br. Res. 86:134-138, 1975.

Kostowski, W., Giacalone, E., Garatinni, S. and Valzelli, L.: Electrical stimulation of midbrain raphe: Biochemical, behavioral and bioelectric effects. European J. Pharmacol. 7:170-175, 1969.

Murphin, D.: A parametric study of the effects of nicotine's discriminative control on tests od dose transfer and time duration for three schedules of reinforcement. Unpublished M.S. Thesis, Virginia Commonwealth University, Richmond, VA., 1974.

Rosecrans, J.A.: Effects of nicotine on behavioral arousal and brain 5-hydroxytryptamine function in female rats selected for differences in activity. European J. Pharmacol. 14:29-37, 1971a.

Rosecrans, J.A.: Effects of nicotine on brain area 5-hydroxytryptamine function in male and female rats separated for differences of activity. European J. Pharmacol. 16:123-137, 1971b.

Rosecrans, J.A.: Brain area nicotine levels in male and female rats with different levels of spontaneous activity. Neuropharmacol. 11:863-870, 1972.

Rosecrans, J.A. and Schechter, M.D.: Brain area nicotine levels in male and female rats of two strains. Arch. Int. Pharmacodyn. 196:46-54, 1972.

Rosecrans, J.A., Dren, A.T. and Domino, E.F.: Effects of physostigmine on rat brain acetylcholine, acetylcholinesterase and conditioned pole jumping Neuropharmacol. 7:127-134, 1968.

Rosecrans, J.A., Goodloe, M.H., Bennett, G.J. and Hirschhorn, I.D.: Morphine as a discriminative cue: Effects of amine depletors and naloxone. European J. Pharmacol. 21:252-256, 1973.

Rosecrans, J.A., Elchisak, M.A. and Schechter, M.D.: Dopamine and psychoactive drug action: A further evaluation. Fed. Proc. 60:506, 1976.

Schechter, M.D. and Rosecrans, J.A.: CNS effect of nicotine as the discriminative stimulus for the rat in a T-maze. Life Sciences 10:821-832, 1971a.

Schechter, M.D. and Rosecrans, J.A.: Behavioral evidence for two types of cholinergic receptors in the CNS. European J. Pharmacol: 15:375-378, 1971b.

Schechter, M.D. and Rosecrans, J.A.: Nicotine as a discriminative cue in rats: Inability of related drugs to produce a nicotine-like cueing effect. Psychopharmacology 27:374-387, 1972a.

Schechter, M.D. and Rosecrans, J.A.: Effect of mecamylamine on discrimination between nicotine- and arecoline-produced cues. European J. Pharmacol. 17:179-182, 1972b.

Schechter, M.D. and Rosecrans, J.A.: Atropine antagonism of arecoline-cued behavior in the rat. Life Science 11:517-523, 1972c.

Schechter, M.D. and Rosecrans, J.A.: Nicotine as a discriminative stimulus in rats depleted of norepinephrine or 5-hydroxytryptamine. Psychopharmacology 24:417-429, 1972d.

Schechter, M.D. and Rosecrans, J.A.: d-Amphetamine as a discriminative cuep Drugs with similar stimulus properties. European J. Pharmacol. 21:212-216, 1973.

Schechter, M.D.: Transfer of state-dependent control of discriminative behavior between subcutaneously and intraventricularly administered nicotine and saline. Psychopharmacology 32:327-335, 1973.

X. ACKNOWLEDGEMENTS

The authors would like to thank the following individuals for their valuable contributions: Drs. M.D. Schechter, I.D. Hirschhorn and R.L. Hayes; Messrs. G. Krynock, M. Spencer, M. Newburn, G. Bennett, P. Hickman; Ms. P. Newlon, J. Harry and D. Murphin. In addition this research could not have been conducted without the generous research support from the Council for Tobacco Research and AMA Education and Research Foundation.

DRUGS AS DISCRIMINABLE EVENTS IN HUMANS

Jack L. Altman
INRS-Santé, Université du Québec
Hôpital L. H. Lafontaine
Montreal, Quebec, Canada

Jean-Marie Albert
Institut de Recherches Psychiatriques de Joliette
Hôpital St-Charles, Joliette, Quebec, Canada

Stephen L. Milstein
INRS-Santé, Université du Québec
Hôpital L. H. Lafontaine
Montreal, Quebec, Canada

Isaac Greenberg
Alcohol and Drug Abuse Research Center
McLean Hospital, Belmont, Massachusetts
U.S.A.

I. INTRODUCTION

Behavioral pharmacology has generally focused upon one aspect of drug action, the unconditioned effect. This usually describes the influence of administered substanced upon either physiological (e.g., heart rate, temperature), behavioral (e.g., latency, discrimination ability), or psychological (e.g., mood, personality) measures (Efron, 1968). It is possible, however, to examine other drug properties. For example, the ability of compounds to function as reinforcers has been demonstrated in studies in which organisms will emit specified behaviors to obtain drugs (Schuster and Thompson, 1969; Brecher, 1972). In addition, there is now widespread evidence derived from the animal laboratory that ingested substances can act as stimulus events (Thompson and Pickens, 1971) controlling behavior in the same way as such traditional stimuli as lights or sounds. The remainder of this chapter will concern itself with the capacity of drugs to function as discriminable events in humans.

II. DRUGS AS DISCRIMINATIVE EVENTS VS STATE-DEPENDENT LEARNING

Research examining drugs as discriminable events has utilized two major procedures: one resulting in a phenomenon known as dissociated or state-dependent learning (SDL); the other, in drug discrimination learning or drugs functioning as discriminative events ($S^{D'}$s) (for good theoretical reviews of this area, see Brown et al., 1968; Barry, 1974; Colpaert et al., 1976). Much confusion has occurred because the two procedures have been treated interchangeably as if they represented the same psychological and pharmacological mechanisms. It is essential to distinguish among behavioral procedures used in pharmacological research since different procedures employing identical compounds and dose levels can produce very different drug effects (Kelleher and Morse, 1968).

A. Drugs as $S^{D'}$s

Discriminative stimuli ($S^{D'}$s) are events which control the occurrence of a response by signalling or indicating when the response is likely to produce consequences. Such cues or $S^{D'}$s control many human behaviors: for example, traffic lights signal the appropriate* driving responses; facial expressions, the appropriate verbal responses; weather conditions, the appropriate "getting-dressed" responses. Employing drugs as $S^{D'}$s, the same stimulus definition applies. Given one drug (or one dose), response A is appropriate and if emitted will produce a consequence; given another drug (or dose), response B is appropriate and if produced will result in the consequence. The only cue signalling the correct behavior is produced by the internal action of the compound ingested. This phenomenon may explain the often excessive behavior of people at cocktail parties. For example, telling an employer "off" or acting sexually aggressive are generally not appropriate behaviors when sober, indeed, they may result in aversive consequences but, in the right setting (i.e., following consumption of alcohol), they occur frequently and are often reinforced.

B. State-Dependent Learning

Apart from controlling specific responses, stimuli can function in a more general manner as well. That is, stimuli forming the

---

*"Appropriate" only in terms of the consequences likely to result from the behavior.

background environment can be shown to alter behavior occurring in that environment if the stimuli are abruptly changed (Bindra, 1959). There is no direct relationship between these "background" stimuli and the behavior as in the case of S^D's, yet sudden shifts in these stimuli will produce shifts in behavior. For example, if subjects are accustomed to working at a certain noise level, a sudden large increase or decrease in the noise will produce a work stoppage. There is no relationship between the background noise and the task, that is, subjects can work adequately and get paid no matter what the noise (or stillness) background is like (within limits, of course), yet a sudden change in the background stimulus can result in a change in behavior. In the same way, drugs may function as background stimuli. Ingested compounds may form a background environment for behaviors occurring in their presence; removing or replacing the drugs (i.e., the background stimuli) will change the background environment and hence affect the behaviors.

III. STATE-DEPENDENT LEARNING IN HUMANS

State-dependent learning (or dissociated learning) has occurred if a behavior learned in the presence of a drug does not appear in the drug's absence. (Conversely, behaviors learned in a non-drug state will not occur in the drugged condition.) The behavior appears to be conditional upon the drug (or non-drug) state present during acquisition, although neither the subjects nor the investigators have established a specific relationship between the drug state and behavior. In general, researchers investigating SDL have employed a 2X2 design (see Overton, 1972 for a good review of SDL procedures) in order to unequivocally demonstrate state-specific effects. Subjects usually undergo an initial training session and are subsequently tested for recall at some later session. Compounds can be administered at both sessions, at neither, or at one and not the other creating 4 possible subject groups: (1) DRUG-DRUG, (2) PLACEBO-PLACEBO, (3) DRUG-PLACEBO, (4) PLACEBO-DRUG. If SDL occurs, recall will be better for groups (1) and (2) than for groups (3) and (4).

Dissociated-learning research in humans has concentrated upon the state-dependent properties of a relatively small number of substances. Table 1 summarizes the available data listing the drugs and tasks employed to test for SDL effects. Among the first reports published were observations of the inability of patients to recall information presented while they were under general anesthesia. However, SDL was not conclusively shown since the investigators did not repeat the anesthetic experience for their patients. Several experimenters (Cheek, 1959; Levinson, 1965) hypnotized their patients at the second session (replacing the

TABLE 1. Drugs and Tasks Tested for Dissociated Learning in Humans.

DRUG	MEASURE	REFERENCES
General anesthetic	Recall of events occurring while under drugs.	Cheek, 1959; Levinson, 1965; Greenberg et al., 1969.
	Recognition of line drawing and recall of letter and word-pairs.	Osborn et al., 1967.
Alcohol	Recall of details during infusion period. Serial-anticipation learning. Verbal learning. Word associations.	Diethelm & Barr, 1962. Storm & Caird, 1967. Goodwin et al., 1969. Goodwin et al., 1969; Weingartner & Faillace, 1971; Goodwin et al., 1974; Crow & Ball, 1975.
	Picture recognition. Avoidance. Paired-associates learning. Word recognition. EEG, skin resistance, respiration, pulse volume, heart rate, finger maze.	Goodwin et al., 1969; Crow & Ball, 1975. Goodwin et al., 1969. Tarter, 1970. Goodwin et al., 1974.
		Crow & Ball, 1975.
Marihuana	Visual avoidance, recall of ordered objects. Verbal learning.	Hill et al., 1973. Hill et al., 1973; Rickels et al., 1973; Cohen & Rickels, 1974; Stillman et al., 1974; Darley et al., 1974; Stillman et al., 1976.

TABLE 1. Drugs and Tasks Tested for Dissociated Learning in Humans.
(CONTINUED)

DRUG	MEASURE	REFERENCES
Marihuana	Recognition of pictures and picture arrangements. Psychomotor tasks.	Stillman et al., 1974. Beautrais & Marks, 1976.
Amphetamine	Recall of nonsense syllables. Recall of geometric shapes. Paired-associates learning.	Bustamante et al., 1968. Bustamante et al., 1970. Hurst et al., 1969; Roffman et al., 1972.
	Finger-maze learning.	Roffman et al., 1972.
Amobarbital	Recall of nonsense syllables. Recall of geometric shapes. Serial, paired-associates, and neologisms learning, pursuit rotor, visual reaction.	Bustamante et al., 1968. Bustamante et al., 1970. Ley et al., 1972.

anesthetic with hypnosis) and did produce some recall. The one experiment to administer the anesthetic (Thiopental) a second time (Osborn et al., 1967) produced results almost completely opposite to those predicted by SDL.

The compound tested most frequently in the dissociated learning procedure has been ethyl alcohol. Like the anesthetics, the original interest in alcohol was generated by clinical reports of non-drugged (i.e., sober) patients forgetting drug-related activities (Diethelm & Barr, 1962; Goodwin, 1974). The experiments with alcohol have produced good evidence for its state-specific effects (Goodwin et al., 1969; Weingartner & Faillace, 1971; Crow & Ball, 1975), although only partially successful (Storm & Caird, 1967; Tarter, 1970) and completely unsuccessful (Goodwin et al., 1974) results have also been reported. Much of the variability in the alcohol studies may have been caused by differences in (1) the subject populations used (i.e., normals vs alcoholics), (2) the dose and type of alcohol administered (e.g., vodka vs gin), or (3) the training procedures employed during the experimental sessions (e.g., the number of trials or items).

We have noted that clinical findings are often responsible for much of the interest in the state-specific effects of compounds. An additional source of interest has been provided by the relationship between the abuse potential of substances and their state-dependent properties (Overton, 1973). In general, there is a direct positive relationship between the degree of dissociation of a drug and the degree to which it is abused. It is primarily this relationship which has led to experiments examining the state dependent properties of marihuana, amphetamine, and amobarbital.

Employing verbal memory tasks, researchers have shown that marihuana produced SDL among "light" cannabis users (Hill et al., 1973; Rickels et al., 1973; Darley et al., 1974; Stillman et al., 1974; 1976). By contrast several teams have failed to demonstrate marihuana-induced SDL. Cohen & Rickels (1974) used "heavy" smokers and a verbal memory task, but found no evidence for SDL. Similarly, Beautrais & Marks (1976) employing a series of psychomotor tasks failed to establish SDL in "light", "moderate", and "heavy" users.

Both positive and negative SDL results have also been obtained with amphetamine (AMP). Bustamante and his co-workers (1968, 1970) found clear dissociated-learning effects; other investigators (Hurst et al., 1969; Roffman et al., 1972) have not. The difference may lie in the quantity of AMP subjects ingested. Bustamante et al., (1968, 1970) administered 20 mg AMP capsules as their standard dose, while the Hurst (1969) and Roffman groups (1972) employed 14 mg/70 kg and 10 mg doses respectively.

Although only a few experiments have examined the state-specific properties of amobarbital, the data are consistent. SDL occurred with 200 mg amobarbital in all the studies carried out thusfar (Bustamante et al., 1968; 1970; Ley et al., 1972).

Reviewing briefly, SDL appears to be a genuine, if not wholly predictable, occurrence in humans. The few compounds tested for state-specific actions have yielded inconsistent results suggesting that many of the significant factors regulating the state dependent mechanism are still unknown. In general, large doses are necessary to ensure the effect, a requirement which will understandably limit inquiry into this phenomenon in man.

IV. DRUGS AS DISCRIMINATIVE EVENTS ($S^{D'}$s) IN HUMANS

To demonstrate the discriminative properties of a drug, individuals must emit one behavior (an "identification" response) in the presence of (i.e., after having ingested) that drug, and another behavior in the presence of another substance. Ideally, the experimental paradigm should include a training procedure in which subjects experience the different compounds and receive explicit consequences (or feedback) after responding. This might reduce some of the variability in the results of experiments investigating the stimulus properties of drugs by (1) attempting to control for the different drug-histories subjects bring into studies, and (2) clarifying both the behaviors required for drug identification and the consequences for those behaviors. Unfortunately, none of the human studies (Table 2) reviewed in this chapter systematically investigated the discriminative properties of compounds in this manner. Much of the available information describing drugs as $S^{D'}$s was generated as a by-product of research which examined other drug effects and therefore did not concern itself with techniques best-suited to test drugs as stimuli. Generally, subjects were simply asked to identify either the specific substance they think they consumed or the drug class to which the substance belongs. Using this indirect approach, investigators collected data describing the discriminative properties of the following drug categories: narcotics, stimulants, hallucinogens, anesthetics, and tranquillizers.

A. Narcotics as $S^{D'}$s

Most of the information concerning the detectability of narcotics has come from the excellent work performed by the Addiction Research Center in Lexington, Kentucky. It is important

TABLE 2. Drugs Tested for Discriminability in Humans (CONTINUED)

DRUG	DOSES (mg)	REFERENCES
diphenoxylate hydrochloride	70 / 70kg	Gorodetzky et al., 1975.
tetrahydroisoquinoline	600 - 1000/70kg	Fraser et al., 1961.
		Fraser et al., 1961.
Hallucinogens		
lysergic acid diethylamide	0.005 - 0.1	Murphree, 1962.
marihuana	variable	Weil et al., 1968; Manno et al., 1970; Jones, 1971; Klonoff, 1973; Milstein et al., 1975 a,b,; Peters et al., 1976.
Anesthetics		
nitrous oxide	30%	Steinberg, 1956.
amobarbital	200	Hawkins et al., 1961.
pentobarbital	50 - 100/70kg	Lasagna et al., 1955.
secobarbital	100 - 200	Goldstone et al., 1958; Hurst et al., 1973.
Tranquillizers		
chlorpromazine	25	Hawkins et al., 1961; Murphree, 1962.
meprobamate	200 - 800	Hawkins et al., 1961; Holliday & Devery, 1961.
chlordiazepoxide	25	Hurst et al., 1973.
Others amitriptyline	25	Holliday & Devery, 1961.
phenoxybenzamine	10 - 30	Murphree, 1962.

TABLE 2. Drugs Tested for Discriminability in Humans

DRUG	DOSES (mg)	REFERENCES
Stimulants		
d-amphetamine	7.5 - 40	Lasagna et al., 1955; Goldstone et al., 1958; Hawkins et al., 1961; Holliday & Devery, 1961; Martin et al., 1970; Hurst et al., 1973; Griffith et al., 1975; Fischman et al., 1976.
dl-amphetamine	14/70kg	Hurst et al., 1973.
d-methamphetamine	15 - 30/70kg	Martin et al., 1970.
ephedrine	75 - 150/70kg	Martin et al., 1970.
phenmetrazine	35 - 70/70kg	Martin et al., 1970.
methylphenidate	15 - 30/70kg	Martin et al., 1970.
dl-fenfluramine	60 - 240	Griffith et al., 1975.
cocaine	4 - 32	Fischman et al., 1976
Narcotics		
morphine	6 - 22.5/70kg	Lasagna et al., 1955; Fraser et al., 1961; Martin & Fraser, 1961; Martin et al., 1965; Jasinski et al., 1970.
diacetylmorphine (heroin)	2 - 8/70 kg	Lasagna et al., 1955; Martin & Fraser, 1961.
codeine	60 - 140/70kg	Fraser et al., 1961.
propoxyphene	300 - 600/70kg	Fraser et al., 1961.
pentazocine	10 - 60/70kg	Jasinski et al., 1970.
nalorphine	8 - 32/70kg	Martin et al., 1965; Jasinski et al., 1970.
cyclazocine	0.5 - 2/70kg	Martin et al., 1965.
naltrexone	0.01 - 200	Martin et al., 1973; Resnick et al., 1974;

to note, however, that the Lexington data are specific to the
particular population tested, primarily, prisoners with extensive
drug histories and may not apply to groups without a similar
drug-abuse background.

The opiates most commonly tested for discriminability have
been morphine, diacetylmorphine or heroin, and nalorphine
(Lasagna et al., 1955; Martin & Fraser, 1961; Martin et al.,
1965; Jasinski et al., 1970). Other substances investigated have
included codeine, propoxyphene, naltrexone, cyclazocine, and
pentazocine (Fraser et al., 1961; Martin et al., 1965; 1973;
Jasinski et al., 1970). (See Table 2 for additional compounds.)
Subjects identified the drug by filling out a "single-dose
questionnaire" in which they could describe the substance ingested
by choosing among the following categories: "blank" (placebo),
"dope" (narcotic analgesic), cocaine, marihuana, "goofball"
(barbiturate), "benny" (dextroamphetamine), others, and
"uncertain". With this procedure, the discrimination threshold
(arbitrarily defined as the drug dose producing correct identification at least 50% of the time) of morphine was found to be
less than 6 mg/70kg. when administered intravenously (Martin
& Fraser, 1961), and about 15 mg/70 kg when injected subcutaneously (Martin et al., 1965; Jasinski et al., 1970). Thresholds
of other opiates were: codeine, 60 mg/70kg. (i.v.) and 140 mg/
70 kg (p.o.); propoxyphene, 120 mg/70 kg. (i.v.) and 600 mg/
70 kg (p.o.) (Martin & Fraser, 1961); heroin, 4 mg/70 kg (i.v.)
(Martin & Fraser, 1961). The opioid antagonists, nalorphine,
cyclazocine, and pentazocine, possessed both narcotic and barbiturate characteristics, (according to the questionnaire) making
threshold determination difficult (Martin et al., 1965; Jasinski
et al., 1970). Naltrexone, on the other hand, a "pure" narcotic
antagonist, was indistinguishable from placebo (Martin et al.,
1973; Gorodetzky et al., 1975) although some agonistic effects
were noted, especially at doses greater than 100 mg (Resnick
et al., 1974).

B. Stimulants as $S^{D'}$s

In general, the experiments examining the discriminative
properties of stimulants offered subjects three identification
choices following drug ingestion: stimulant, depressant or
sedative, and placebo. The results from the eight studies
reviewed (see Table 2) are remarkably consistent. Except for
one study (Holliday & Devery, 1961) which employed fatigued
students as subjects, the discriminability of amphetamine was
very low. Dose levels of less than 20 mg were either
indistinguishable from placebo (Goldstone et al., 1958) or
discriminated from other substances no more than 30% of the
time (Hawkins et al., 1961; Hurst et al., 1973). Administering
20 - 40 mg AMP resulted in better detectability (64%) in some

studies (Griffith et al., 1975), but only marginal improvement (40%) in others (Lasagna et al., 1955; Martin et al., 1970). The detectability of such other stimulants as methamphetamine, methylphenidate and fenfluramine was equally poor (Martin et al., 1970; Griffith et al., 1975).

Two major factors may have been responsible for the poor detection performance of subjects given stimulants: (1) almost all the subjects were students with little drug experience, and (2) they were presented with too many categories as identification choices. The first explanation is not substantiated by the experimental results. The performance of experienced drug users (prisoners) was no different from the students (Lasagna et al., 1955; Martin et al., 1970). The second explanation is more tenable (although why three choices should prove difficult for stimulants and not narcotics is puzzling). When subjects were told that they would be receiving either a stimulant or placebo, they had no difficulty discriminating between AMP and placebo, even at 10 mg doses (Hurst et al., 1973; Fischman et al., 1976).

C. Hallucinogens as $S^{D'}$s

While evaluating the effectiveness of certain agents antagonizing LSD, Murphree (1962) simultaneously examined the stimulus characteristics of all the compounds involved. To ensure familiarity with the action of LSD, Murphree pretreated his subjects with weekly doses of 0.025 - 0.1 mg LSD before he began threshold determination. Subsequent testing with much lower doses (0.005 - 0.025 mg) established that the LSD detection threshold was approximately 0.02 mg, a value much lower than is known to produce hallucinogenic activity (Hoffer & Osmond 1967).

In contrast to the LSD results, the literature dealing with marihuana as an S^D is much more extensive and confusing. Basically, it is unclear whether or not subjects can discriminate between cigarettes containing and cigarettes lacking Δ^9 - THC (the active ingredient of cannabis). An additional factor complicating the discrimination is the type of subject employed, "heavy" or "light" smokers. To date, the experimental results have exhausted all possible outcomes. Researchers have demonstrated that (1) all subjects can easily tell marihuana from placebo (Jones 1971; Milstein et al., 1975a; Peters et al., 1976); (2) subjects have great difficulty distinguishing marihuana from placebo (Manno et al., 1970; Jones, 1971; Klonoff, 1973); (3) "experienced" users are better at detecting the presence of marihuana than inexperienced smokers (Weil et al., 1968;

Milstein, et al., 1975b); and (4) infrequent smokers are better at detecting marihuana than frequent users (Jones, 1971). Contributing to this hodgepodge are such variables as dose, quantity absorbed, expectancy or set, and drug history (Jones, 1971; Nahas, 1973; Klonoff, 1973).

D. Other compounds as $S^{D'}$s

Anesthetics function as very effective $S^{D'}$s. A 200 mg dose of secobarbital, for example, produced 97% correct detection among subjects (Goldstone et al., 1958), while 50 and 100 mg doses of pentobarbital resulted in 100% detection (Lasagna et al., 1955). Less accurate discrimination has also been reported, but this was most probably due to the low level of drug administered or the very specific identification required (Hurst et al., 1973; Hawkins et al., 1961). General anesthetics such as nitrous oxide have also been shown to be potent discriminative events (Steinberg, 1956).

The data describing the discriminative properties of tranquillizers are inconclusive. For example, subjects have both easily discriminated (Hawkins et al., 1961) and have failed to detect (Murphree, 1962) the presence of 25 mg chlorpromazine (CPZ). A high dose of meprobamate (800 mg) had clear S^D properties (Holliday & Devery, 1961); a low dose (200 mg) did not (Hawkins et al., 1961). The only minor tranquillizer tested, 25 mg chlordiazepoxide, was a poor S^D being identified as often as a depressant and placebo as a tranquillizer (Hurst et al., 1973).

In reviewing drugs as $S^{D'}$s, it is apparent that some substances have marked discriminative properties, but that many (up to now) do not. Some of the problems associated with demonstrating drugs as $S^{D'}$s were mentioned earlier in the chapter: subjects were rarely trained in the identification procedure; subjects brought varying degrees of drug experience into the experiment; familiarity with the experimental drugs was not established; the experiments themselves were designed to test hypotheses having little to do with the stimulus properties of compounds. Thus, at this point, we cannot conclude that stimulants (for example) or tranquillizers have few discriminative characteristics. We do not know. What is needed is not only more research in this area, but research appropriate to discovering the S^D properties of drugs. In the following section, we shall describe a pilot experiment which tested directly the discriminative properties of ethanol and diazepam.

V. THE S^D PROPERTIES OF ETHANOL AND DIAZEPAM: A SINGLE-DOSE STUDY

The experiment was designed to investigate the S^D properties of single doses of ethanol and diazepam. Since (for reasons of safety) subjects were not permitted to leave for at least 2 hours following drug ingestion, we decided to simultaneously determine the effects of these compounds upon human operant performance.

A. Materials and Methods

The subjects were 4 females (C.B., N.B., R.B., A.L.) between 30 and 45 years in age and weighing between 50 and 67 kg. Physical and psychiatric examinations prior to the start of the experiment revealed no abnormalities. Before signing an informed consent form agreeing to participate in the experiment, subjects were told that they would be receiving only one substance during the study, either 1-1/2 oz. (45 ml) 94% ethanol or 5 mg diazepam, that the experiment would last a maximum of 10 weekdays, that there was a 50% probability of a subject ingesting drug (or placebo) on any experimental day, and that they would earn a minimum of $100 and a maximum of $150 if they completed the 10 sessions. Subjects were free to terminate their participation at any time retaining whatever money had been earned to that date. On experimental days subjects were asked to abstain from all substances during the 6 hr. before testing.

The subjects were tested in a sound-shielded room containing a chair and table upon which had been placed the experimental apparatus. The apparatus was a wooden console which contained 2 levers (depression of which activated a microswitch), 3 lights (amber, red, green), and a coin dispenser which dispensed tokens worth $.25. The electromechanical devices used to program and record the experimental task requirements, responses, and reinforcers were placed in an adjoining room.

The subjects arrived 15 min. apart starting at 5:00 PM each weekday, and after a check of vital signs received drug or placebo. Two subjects (N.B., A.L.) received either 45 ml. 94% ethanol diluted in 450 ml. orange juice or placebo (450 ml. orange juice with a 3 ml. supernatant layer of ethanol). The remaining 2 subjects (C.B., R.B.) were given either 5 mg diazepam or a placebo pill. In addition, each day, the "diazepam" subjects received the ethanol placebo, and the "ethanol" subjects the diazepam placebo to permit the blind administration of both ethanol and diazepam to all subjects. The experimental session began 60 min. after substance administration.

At the start of each session, the amber light was illuminated and remained on for the duration of the 15 min. session. In the presence of the green light, subjects earned $.25 for every 125 presses on the correct lever (FR 125); in the presence of the red light, subjects were reinforced for holding the correct lever down for 30-33 sec. [differential reinforcement of response duration or DRRD 30 LH 3 (Altman, in press)], release of the manipulandum before 30 sec. or after 33 sec. reset the timing interval. Which lever was correct depended upon the substance consumed by the subject: for 2 subjects the left lever was correct on days drug had been administered and the right lever correct on days placebo had been given, while the reverse was true for the other 2 subjects. Responding upon the incorrect lever had no programmed consequences. Subjects were told that one manipulandum was correct following drug administration, and the other after placebo. Only the first 125 responses of each session served as a measure of drug discriminability since the occurrence or non-occurrence of the first reinforcer functioned as a cue as to which lever was correct. Subjects earned a $7.00 bonus if they selected the correct lever for the session's first 125 responses. During each session the red and green lights were presented in a 50% random probability sequence except that the FR 125 requirement (i.e., the green light) always started the session.

The subjects were initially given 3 days training in the multiple schedule of reinforcement procedure (mult. FR 125 DRRD 30 LH 3) followed by a minimum of 6 consecutive days of random drug or placebo presentation. The random drug-placebo sequence was continued beyond 6 days for those subjects who did not learn to discriminate between drug and placebo to criterion. Criterion was established as 5 consecutive days of correct lever selection since this represented about a 3% probability that subjects could have selected the correct lever by guessing.

C. Results and Discussion

Subjects easily discriminated ethanol from placebo reaching criterion within 6 days. Distinguishing diazepam from placebo proved to be more difficult. One subject (R.B.) learned the discrimination after 8 days, while the other subject (C.B.) continued to lever select at the chance level after 10 days.

Due to the small number of subjects and the single doses

used, we cannot describe confidently the effects of the compounds
upon operant performance. There did not appear to be any
change in FR responding, but we did observe shifts in timing
behavior. Following drug administration, timing accuracy
<u>improved</u> in 3 subjects (C.B., R.B., A.L.) and deteriorated
in one (N.B.). The most significant difference between the
subjects with drug-improved performance and subject N.B.
whose responding was adversely affected by ethanol was the
presence of a nicotine dependence. Subject N.B. was not a
cigarette smoker while the others regularly consumed between
25 and 40 cigarettes per day.

While much of the data collected in this study are tentative
due to the few subjects participating, we feel that this experimental procedure is extremely valuable and productive supplying
information about drug discriminability and the effects of
compounds upon behavior. Current research is concentrating
upon establishing precise dose-response relationships between
the quantity of drug ingested and drug discriminability and
determining the discriminability of other compounds employing
both the present drug-placebo techniques and a drug-drug
paradigm.

VI. CONCLUDING REMARKS

The phenomenon of drugs acting as discriminable events may
result in several significant applications in humans. The first
is the possibility of finding differences between normal and
clinical populations in their sensitivity to drugs. For example,
alcoholics may have different detection thresholds for certain
compounds than non-alcoholics, and investigators might then
examine (for example) specific biological mechanisms in order
to trace the factors responsible for the difference.

A similar line of research might demonstrate differences
in drug sensitivity thresholds between patients with severe
psychological disturbances and normal populations (Greenwood
et al., 1974). Such differences might help in the development
of effective diagnostic techniques. Another important application
might involve teaching individuals to discriminate the S^D
properties of compounds. Clinical populations occasionally
develop side-effects due to the quantities of psychoactive
substances they consume during the course of chemotherapy.
Perhaps patients trained to detect the presence of drugs can
achieve the same therapeutic benefit from low drug levels (thereby eliminating some of the risks of side-effects) as non-trained
patients can from moderate to high doses.

The results of experiments dealing with drugs as S^D's may also cause changes in the classificatory systems describing drugs. Researchers may be able to categorize all psychoactive compounds according to their discriminative properties. That is, they may be able to create "subjective" profiles of drugs using objective techniques. This would also enable investigators to predict into what "subjective" categories newly synthesized compounds would fit. In fact, Overton (1973) has already suggested that a drug's discriminable characteristics might predict its abuse potential.

Finally, the capacity of drugs to function as S^D's might be utilized in traditional psychopharmacological experiments as well. For example researchers could relate the onset (or duration) of drug discriminability to other drug effects -- biochemical, physiological or behavioral. Or, pharmacologists could test the effectiveness of antagonists or blocking agents by preadministering the antagonist and determining whether the blocked compound still retained its S^D properties.

REFERENCES

ALTMAN, J.L.: Drugs and the production of temporal intervals in the rat. Prog. Neuropsychopharmacol., in press.

BARRY, H.: III: Classification of drugs according to their discriminable effects in rats. Fed. Proc. 33: 1814-1824, 1974.

BEAUTRAIS, A.L. and MARKS, D.F.: A test of state dependency effects in marihuana intoxication for the learning of psychomotor tasks. Psychopharmacologia 46: 37-40, 1976.

BINDRA, D.: Stimulus change reactions to novelty and response decrement. Psychol. Rev. 66: 96-103, 1959.

BRECHER, E.M.: Licit and illicit drugs. Consumer's Union, Mt. Vernon, New York, 1972.

BROWN, A., FELDMAN, R.S. and MOORE, J.W.: Conditional discrimination learning based upon chlordiazepoxide: Dissociation or cue? J. Comp. Physiol. Psychol. 66: 211-215, 1968.

BUSTAMANTE, J.A., ROSSELLO, A., JORDAN, A., PRADERA, E. and INSUA, A.: Learning and drugs. Physiol. Behav. 3: 553-555, 1968.

BUSTAMANTE, J.A., JORDAN, A., VILA, M., GONZALEZ, A. and INSUA, A.: State dependent learning in humans. Physiol. Behav. 5: 793-796, 1970.

CHEEK, D.B.: Unconscious perception of meaningful sounds during surgical anesthesia as revealed under hypnosis. Am. J. Clin. Hyp. 1: 101-113, 1959.

COHEN, M.J. and RICKELS, W.H.Jr.: Performance on a verbal learning task by subjects of heavy past marijuana usage. Psychopharmacologia 37: 323-330, 1974.

COLPAERT, F.C., NIEMEGEERS, C.J.E. and JANSSEN, P.A.J.: Theoretical and methodological considerations on drug discrimination learning. Psychopharmacologia 46: 169-177, 1976.

CROW, L.T. and BALL, C.: Alcohol state-dependency and autonomic reactivity. Psychophysiol. 12: 702-706, 1975.

DARLEY, C.F., TINKLENBERG, J.R., ROTH, W.T. and ATKINSON, R.C.: The nature of storage deficits and state-dependent retrieval under marihuana. Psychopharmacologia 37: 139-149, 1974.

DIETHELM, O. and BARR, R.M.: Experimental study of amnesic periods in acute alcohol intoxication. Psychiat. Neurol. 144: 5-14, 1962.

EFRON, D.H.: Psychopharmacology: A review of progress, 1957-1967. U.S. Government Printing Office, Washington, D.C., 1968.

FISCHMAN, M.W., SCHUSTER, C.R., RESNEKOV, L., SHICK, J.F.E., KRASNEGOR, N.A., FENNELL, W. and FREEDMAN, D.X.: Cardiovascular and subjective effects of intravenous cocaine administration in humans. Arch. Gen. Psychiat. 33: 983-989, 1976.

FRASER, H.F., VAN HORN, G.D., MARTIN, W.R., WOLBACH, A.B. and ISBELL, H.: Methods for evaluating addiction liability. (A) "Attitude" of opiate addicts toward opiate-like drugs; (B) A short-term "direct" addiction test. J. Pharmacol. Exp. Ther. 133: 371-387, 1961.

GOLDSTONE, S., BOARDMAN, W.K. and LHAMON, W.T.: Effect of quinal barbitone, dextro-amphetamine, and placebo on apparent time. Br. J. Psychol. 49: 324-328, 1958.

GOODWIN, D.W.: Alcoholic blackout and state-dependent learning. Fed. Proc. 33: 1833-1835, 1974.

GOODWIN, D.W., POWELL, B., BREMER, D., HOINE, H. and STERN, J.: Alcohol and recall: State-dependent effects in man. Science 163: 1358-1360, 1969.

GOODWIN, D.W., POWELL, B., HILL, S.Y., LIEBERMAN, W. and VIAMONTES, J.: Effects of alcohol on "dissociated" learning in alcoholics. J. Nerv. Ment. Dis. 158: 198-201, 1974.

GORODETZKY, C.W., MARTIN, W.R., JASINSKI, D.R., MANSKY, P.A. and CONE, E.J.: Human pharmacology of naltrexone. In: Developments in the Field of Drug Abuse, ed. by E. Senay, V. Shorty and H. Alksne, pp. 749-753, Schenkman Publishing Co., Cambridge, Mass., 1975.

GREENWOOD, M.H., FRIEDEL, J., BOND, A.J., CURZON, G. and LADER, M.H.:

The acute effects of intravenous infusion of L-tryptophan in normal subjects. Clin. Pharmacol. Ther. 16: 455-464, 1974.

GRIFFITH, J.D., NUTT, J.G. and JASINSKI, D.R.: A comparison of fenfluramine and amphetamine in man. Clin. Pharmacol. Ther. 18: 563-570, 1975.

HAWKINS, D.R., PACE, R., PASTERNACK, B. and SANDIFER, M.G.Jr.: A multivariant psychopharmacologic study in normals. Psychosom. Med. 23: 1-17, 1961.

HILL, S.Y., SCHWIN, R., POWELL, B. and GOODWIN, D.W.: State-dependent effects of marihuana on human memory. Nature 243: 241-242, 1973.

HOFFER, A. and OSMOND, H.: The Hallucinogens, Academic Press, New York, 1967.

HOLLIDAY, A.R. and DEVERY, W.J.: Effects of drugs on the performance of a task by fatigued subjects. Clin. Pharmacol. Ther. 3: 5-15, 1961.

HURST, P.M., RADLOW, R., CHUBB, N.C. and BAGLEY, S.K.: Effects of d-amphetamine on acquisition, persistence, and recall. Am. J. Psychol. 82: 307-319, 1969.

HURST, P.M., WEIDNER, M.F., RADLOW, R. and ROSS, S.: Drugs and placebos: Drug guessing by normal volunteers. Psychol. Rep. 33: 683-694, 1973.

JASINSKI, D.R., MARTIN, W.R. and HOELDTKE, R.D.: Effects of short-and long-term administration of pentazocine in man. Clin. Pharmacol. Ther. 11: 385-403, 1970.

JONES, R.T.: Marihuana-induced "high": Influence of expectation, setting and previous drug experience. Pharmacol. Rev. 23: 359-369, 1970.

KELLEHER, R.T. and MORSE, W.H.: Determinants of the specificity of behavioral effects of drugs. Ergebnisse der Physiologie 60: 1-56, 1968.

KLONOFF, H.: Strategy and tactics of marijuana research. Can. Med. Assoc. J. 108: 145-150, 1973.

LASAGNA, L., Von FELSINGER, J.M. and BEECHER, H.K.: Drug-induced mood changes in man. JAMA 157: 1006-1020, 1955.

LEVINSON, B.W.: States of awareness during general anesthesia. Br. J. Anesth. 37: 544-546, 1965.

LEY, P., JAIN, V.K., SWINSON, R.P., EAVES, D., BRADSHAW, P.W., KINCEY, J.A., CROWDER, R. and ABBISS, S.: A state-dependent learning effect produced by amylobarbitone sodium. Br. J. Psychiat. 120: 511-515, 1972.

MANNO, J.E., KIPLINGER, G.R., BENNET, I.F., HAINES, S. and FORNEY, R.B.: Comparative effects of smoking marihuana or placebo on human motor and mental performance. Clin. Pharmacol. Ther. 11: 808-815, 1970.

MARTIN, W.R. and FRASER, H.F.: A comparative study of physiological and subjective effects of heroin and morphine administered intravenously in postaddicts. J. Pharmacol. Exp. Ther. 133: 388-399, 1961.

MARTIN, W.R., FRASER, H.F., GORODETZKY, C.W. and ROSENBERG, D.E.: Studies of the dependence-producing potential of the narcotic antagonist 2-cyclopropylmethyl-2'-hydroxy-5,9-dimethyl-6,7-benzomorphan (cyclazocine, WIN-20,740, ARC II-C-3). J. Pharmacol. Exp. Ther. 150: 426-436, 1965.

MARTIN, W.R., SLOAN, J.W., SAPIRA, J.D. and JASINSKI, D.R.: Physiologic, subjective, and behavioral effects of amphetamine, methamphetamine, ephedrine, phenmetrazine, and methylphenidate in man. Clin. Pharmacol. Ther. 12: 245-247, 1970.

MARTIN, W.R., JASINSKI, D.R. and MANSKY, P.A.: Naltrexone, an antagonist for the treatment of heroin dependence. Arch. Gen. Psychiat. 28: 784-791, 1973.

MILSTEIN, S.L., MACCANNELL, K., KARR, G. and CLARK, S.: Marijuana-produced impairments in coordination. J. Nerv. Ment. Dis. 161: 26-31, 1975a.

MILSTEIN, S.L., MACCANNELL, K., KARR, G. and CLARK, S.: Marijuana-produced changes in pain tolerance: Experienced and non-experienced subjects. Int. Pharmacopsychiat. 10: 177-182, 1975b.

MURPHREE, H.B.: Quantitative studies in humans on the antagonism of lysergic acid diethylamide by chlorpromazine and phenoxybenzamine. Clin. Pharmacol. Ther. 3: 314-320, 1962.

NAHAS, G.G.: Clinical pharmacology of cannabis sativa with special reference to delta-9-THC. Bull. Narcot. 25: 9-39, 1973.

OSBORN, A.G., BUNKER, J.P., COOPER, L.M., FRANK, G.S. and HILGARD, E.R.: Effects of thiopental sedation on learning and memory. Science 157: 574-576, 1967.

OVERTON, D.A.: State-dependent learning produced by alcohol and its relevance to alcoholism. In: The Biology of Alcoholism, vol. 2, Physiology and Behavior, ed. by B. Kissin and H. Begleiter, pp. 193-217, Plenum Press, New York, 1972.

OVERTON, D.A.: State-dependent learning produced by addicting drugs. In: Opiate Addiction: Origins and Treatment, ed. by S. Fisher and A.M. Freedman, pp. 61-75, Winston & Sons, Washington, D.C., 1973.

PETERS, B.S., LEWIS, E.G., DUSTMAN, R.E., STRAIGHT, R.C. and BECK, E.

C.: Sensory, perceptual, motor and cognitive functioning and subjective reports following oral administration of Δ^9-tetrahydrocannabinol. Psychopharmacology 47: 141-148, 1976.

RESNICK, R.B., VOLAVKA, J., FREEDMAN, A.M. and THOMAS, M.: Studies of EN-1639A (Naltrexone): A new narcotic antagonist. Am. J. Psychiat. 131: 646-650, 1974.

RICKELS, W.H.Jr., COHEN, M.J., WHITAKER, C.A. and McINTYRE, K.E.: Marijuana induced state-dependent verbal learning. Psychopharmacologia 30: 349-354, 1973.

ROFFMAN, M., MARSHALL, P., SILVERSTEIN, A., KARKALAS, J., SMITH, N. and LAL, H.: Failure to demonstrate "amphetamine state" controlling learned behavior in humans. In: Drug Addiction: Clinical and Socio-legal Aspects, vol. 2, ed. by J.M. Singh, L. Miller and H. LAL, pp. 53-57, Futura Publishing, Mt. Kisco, New York, 1972.

SCHUSTER, C.R. and THOMPSON, T.: Self-administration of and behavioral dependence on drugs. Annu. Rev. Pharmacol. 9: 483-502, 1969.

STEINBERG, H.: "Abnormal behaviour" induced by nitrous oxide. Br. J. Psychol. 47: 183-194, 1956.

STILLMAN, R.C., WEINGARTNER, H., WYATT, R.J., GILLIN, J.C. and EICH, J.: State-dependent (dissociative) effects of marihuana on human memory. Arch. Gen. Psychiat. 31: 81-85, 1974.

STILLMAN, R.C., EICH, J.E., WEINGARTNER, H. and WYATT, R.J.: Marihuana-induced state-dependent amnesia and its reversal by cueing. In: The Pharmacology of Marihuana, ed. by M.C. Braude and S. Szara, pp. 453-456, Raven Press, New York, 1976.

STORM, T. and CAIRD, W.K.: The effects of alcohol on serial verbal learning in chronic alcoholics. Psychon. Sci. 9: 43-44, 1967.

TARTER, R.E.: Dissociate effects of ethyl alcohol. Psychon. Sci. 20: 342-343, 1970.

THOMPSON, T. and PICKENS, R.: Stimulus Properties of Drugs, Appleton Century Crofts, New York, 1971.

WEIL, A.T., ZINBERG, N.E. and NELSEN, J.M.: Clinical and Psychological effects of marijuana in man. Science 162: 1234-1242, 1968.

WEINGARTNER, H. and FAILLACE, L.A.: Alcohol state-dependent learning in man. J. Nerv. Ment. Dis. 153: 395-406, 1971.

DRUG INDUCED DISCRIMINABLE STIMULI:
PAST RESEARCH AND FUTURE PERSPECTIVES

Harbans Lal

Department of Pharmacology & Toxicology
and
Department of Psychology
University of Rhode Island
Kingston, R.I. 02881

I. DRUGS AS DISCRIMINATIVE STIMULI

A. Properties of Drugs

Stimuli are conventionally defined as environmental events that reliably control behaviors. The rate of behavioral emission is different in the presence of certain stimuli than in their absence. The experimental characterization of a stimulus is exclusively based upon the behaviors that are either emitted or elicited in the presence of the stimulus. The type of functional relationship between a stimulus and a response determines a stimulus category. At present many stimulus categories are recognized (for discussion see Thompson and Pickens, 1971).

Usually stimuli consist of changes in the physical environment such as changes in the visual and auditory energy patterns. Therefore, until recently, events occurring only in the external environment were recognized as stimuli, even though it was assumed that external events act as stimuli through the sensory apparatus located within the organism. With the availability of drugs as research tools and advancing technology in psychopharmacology research, it is now realized that there are many events occurring within the body that can also act as stimuli. By now many drug actions are known to possess stimulus properties (for review see Thompson and Pickens, 1971). As a result of these developments the conventional definition of the term stimulus needs to be modified to include as stimuli, events that are primarily initiated within the body of an organism.

Although drugs produce many types of stimuli, the present discussion will be limited only to the drug-induced discriminative stimuli. Discriminative stimuli (DS) are physical or biological events which reliably control behaviors that occur in their presence or immediately following them. A response is reinforced in the presence of a DS and not in its absence. Where two alternating stimuli are employed one response is reinforced in the presence of one stimulus and a different response is reinforced in the presence of the second stimulus. Since the animal makes differential responses to unlike stimuli, a discrimination process is inferred. Also, because the response selection must be based upon a reliable perception of the stimulus sensation, the resulting differential responses are taken as a reliable measure of the stimulus perception.

It is now realized that whenever the nervous system is excited through a stimulus, a new state is organized within the nervous system and certain components of that state are perceived, some dominantly and others minimally. In the beginning, the organism responds to the dominant cue within the stimulus complex. The other cues are effectively ignored as irrelevant at that time. Subsequently, if the dominant cue is found reliably associated with the response-consequences, it is adopted for discrimination learning. However, if a reliable association is not found, one of the other cues is selected.

During drug discrimination learning, the animal does not respond to the drug cue in the beginning. Rather, the subject first responds to other more dominant cues present in its environment. The obvious ones include position of the operandum, sequence of the training sessions, or many other sensory cues because these have been previously relevant for most organisms in their natural environment. Only when these other cues don't work does the distinct stimulus associated with the drug action become dominant. From the data available in the acquisition experiments it is often seen that if the drug stimulus is presented concurrently with other discriminable stimuli, the laboratory animals first ignore the drug cues and attend to other physical cues. It is only when the external cues are made irrelevant to differential reinforcement that the drug cues are learned.

As drugs can also produce eliciting stimuli, if the experimental design is not properly controlled, the eliciting stimuli may be confused with the DS. In the case of an eliciting stimulus, a response is elicited immediately, and often reflexively, after the presentation of a stimulus. A tone (Miksic et al., 1975) or odor (Lal et al., 1976), for example, which does not originally elicit hyperthermia, will do so after it has been paired with injections of morphine that are hyperthermic. In contrast, a stimulus functions as a DS if it "sets the occasion" for the occurrance of a response. These two types of stimuli can be distinguished experimentally. In experimental situations in which only one response is allowed to occur, it is hard to distinguish between the two types of stimuli. However, by using a free operant design the eliciting and discriminative properties of a stimulus can be very well distinguished. According to this design, continued emmission of responses is required in the case of discriminative responding. As long as the stimulus is present responses will be emitted either at some steady rate or in temporal pattern that is characteristic of the schedule of reinforcement. Thus, once the drug-stimulus is provided, it is followed by an indefinite number of responses which are terminated either by the onset of satiation or by the removal of the stimulus.

B. Acquisition of Discriminative Control

It is evident from many experiments reported elsewhere in this book that differential reinforcement is necessary for the establishment of a stimulus control by drugs. Although it is feasible to establish the stimulus control of a drug by simply reinforcing one operant repeatedly in the presence of the drug action as DS, this approach is cumbersome and needs a large number of sessions with several control groups in order to establish that the stimulus control by drugs has been acquired. A better way is to establish within-animal discrimination. This is best done by differentially reinforcing two responses. The organism is allowed to emit two different responses but only one is reinforced in the presence of the drug stimulus. The alternate response is reinforced in the presence of another drug or a placebo. This has been proven to be the most effective experimental procedure reported to date. This type of procedure is decidedly superior to the use of the state-dependent-learning paradigm where only one response is allowed to occur. By differential reinforcement the stimulus control of a drug is acquired after a response has already been learned. In contrast, in the state-dependent paradigm a response must be learned only in the presence of the drug.

After stimulus control of a drug action is acquired, it can be further sharpened by a variety of methods. It is assumed that usually the discriminative control obtained through the use of drugs does not approach the limits of the discrimination capacity of the organism. Therefore, a finer degree of discrimination between the action of a drug and vehicle can usually be produced by gradually reducing the dosage used. For example, whereas Holtzman (personal communication) found it to be impossible to train rats to discriminate between saline and morphine in a dose of 0.3 mg/kg, he could accomplish this very well in rats who were first trained to discriminate larger doses of morphine from saline. The morphine dose was then gradually reduced and a discrimination between doses of 0 and 0.3 mg/kg was readily achieved.

The other approach to sharpen the drug discrimination is to increase the contrast between the drug action and placebo by providing a sharply contrasting background. For example, usual doses of haloperidol exert very weak stimulus control. However, haloperidol is very easily discriminated in the presence of amphetamine (Weissman, 1976), the presence of which sharpens the perception of the action of haloperidol.

C. Attention and Drug Discrimination

Among sensory psychologists, it is generally recognized that subjects first attend to the stimulus before responding to it. This attention process is variously described as observing, preparatory or orienting responses. An observing response is defined as a response that is emitted before the opportunity for discriminative responding is made available.

Obviously the generalization of an attention hypothesis to drug discrimination is difficult at present. The original hypothesis is derived out of experimental paradigms in which discriminable stimuli lie in the external environment and attending to them by the organisms can be readily observed. In contrast, drug stimuli are produced exclusively within the organism and the attending response to those stimuli will be difficult to observe. However, some investigators do take the "attention" process into account by incorporating an observing response in their experimental paradigm. For example, Shannon and Holtzman (1976) required their subjects to emit an observing response before an opportunity for discriminative responding was made available.

The observing response is an experimental indicator of attention which is still a mentalistic concept. This response is considered to have the function of placing the organism in contact with a discriminative stimulus, a function which is closely identified with the attention process. Although mentalistically it may be felt that the opportunity to focus "attention" will facilitate performance of discriminative tests, it is yet too early to present data which can experimentally verify this concept.

II. NATURE OF DRUG STIMULUS

A. Simulation of Sensory Sensations

Conventional stimuli that are usually made up of environmental events are understood to exert their stimulus properties through stimulation of the sensory mechanisms such as seeing, hearing, olfaction, taste and proprioception. These sensory stimuli originate at peripheral sites which receive the stimulus and are then carried through specific neuronal pathways eventually to be perceived as specific sensations in the higher brain centers. When drug stimuli were originally recognized, they were thought to be the result of a drug action simulating sensory mechanisms. It is true that drugs as chemical substances cause distinct physiological and/or biochemical changes in the body which are capable of stimulating sensory modalities. This stimulation can be considered to provide sensations which are equivalent to the physiological stimulation of receptor mechanisms as are usually provided by physical stimuli. However, there is no evidence as yet available to substantiate this explanation of the DS produced by drugs. As a matter of fact, no known sensory stimulation can be substituted for a drug stimulus in a discrimination task.

Rats trained to discriminate either morphine from saline or pentobarbital from saline fail to emit drug appropriate responses when exposed to the odor of anise oil, a sound, light, darkness, touch, changes in body position to simulate proprioception, or exposure to a variety of social experiences (Miksic and Lal, unpublished data). Although all of the possible sensory experiences can not be tested, there is no indication that the sensory stimuli that have been tested provide even the weakest equivalent of the drug stimulus discriminable by the rats. As a matter of fact, it is known that drugs producing only peripheral actions are harder to discriminate than centrally acting drugs as is illustrated with use of loperamide discussed elsewhere in this book.

B. Modification of Sensory Input

Because of the potent actions produced by the drugs on sensory mechanisms, it is conceivable that the drugs produce discriminable stimuli by distorting the usual nature of sensory experiences. Drug induced hallucinations may be a good example. As the drugs which are known for their hallucination producing properties are well discriminated, it may be said that these drugs produce a specific change in which a certain sensory illusion due to distortion of normal sensory input is perceived and that altered sensory experience constitutes the physiological substate of the DS. There

are a number of experiments which can be cited both to support
or to negate this view at this time. Therefore, additional
research is needed before the role of sensory modification by
drugs in the formation of DS can be critically evaluated.

C. Drug Specific Sensations

Drug actions are more likely to produce their own drug-
specific changes in the CNS which, themselves, constitute specific
sensations. We believe that these changes are qualitatively
different than the conventional sensory experiences and are often
characteristics of a drug class. This aspect will be discussed
at length elsewhere in this chapter and other chapters of the book.
Here it may be sufficient to say that the drugs are capable of
initiating physiological changes in the CNS which are perceived
as unlike those produced by normal life processes. Although, it
is conceivable that the drug action on sensory apparatus can provide a stimulus capable of being discriminated under appropriate
experimental conditions, they are not the usual DS which are
basis for drug discrimination.

D. Contrasts with External Stimuli

External stimuli such as sound, light and pressure are known
to provide discriminative input and so are the internal stimuli
such as drug actions. Data on the similarities and the contrasts
between these two classes of stimuli are not available to any
great extent. However, a few observations can be presented.

An important characteristic of external stimuli is their
alterability (Barry, 1974). An environmental event can be initiated, modified and terminated with great rapidity and precision.
They can either be altered by physical manipulations of the
environment by the experimenter or by modifying their input into
the organism through a selective act of organism itself such as
turning toward or away from the stimulus source. Since the discriminative response is almost always associated with onset,
cessation, or other changes in the characteristics of the external
stimuli, its strength can be easily varied by altering the stimulus.
Secondly, at the intensities usually used, the external stimuli,
possess weak motivational properties. They are often important
only as signals. Therefore the organism can learn to ignore
them when they remain unchanged for a prolonged period.

In contrast to the external stimuli, drug effects have gradual
onset and gradual termination. Here, the transition between non-
drug condition and a drug condition is usually less clear, even
though the fully established drug action provides a strong and

stable stimulus. Also, the drug stimuli can often be considered to possess strong motivational properties because they are often pleasurable or aversive in nature as far as it is known.

The importance of the above mentioned differences between the two stimulus classes has not been studied experimentally. This is because it is not easy to initiate and terminate the drug action by the usual manipulations. Even the use of the intravenous route of administration, the fastest available, provides only an approximation to the control of external stimuli. However, what can be indirectly inferred from the meager data available is that there is a striking similarity between the behavioral properties of both types of stimuli. Thus far there is no known exception. Inspite of different times of onset and their definite pharmacokinetic properties, a given drug is responded to in the same way quite independent of the route of administration as long as time and dose of injections are appropriately adjusted to provide above-threshold strength of action. This suggests that the animals do not attend to the time-response relationship of the drug action as long as a threshold concentration is assured. But rather that they discriminate the mere presence of the drug action.

Whereas the external stimuli are usually considered to involve one channel of input, the number of input channels used by the drug actions to produce a perceivable stimulus is not known. In view of the multiplicity of the effects which most drugs produce it seems likely that the input is more complex than with the external stimuli. Many more experiments will be required to understand the role of this complexity.

Drug produced stimuli impose an inescapable stimulus condition to the organism which may initiate compensatory mechanisms within the animals. Whereas in many cases the direct action of drugs is considered to provide the DS, there may be other instances in which it is the opposite compensatory action which provides that stimulus. Previously, the compensatory mechanism of drug action has been reported to become a conditional response (Roffman and Lal, 1974).

Besides triggering of compensatory changes, the continuous availability of the stimulus provided by a drug may ensure more sustained control of behavior. In this sense the behavioral control exerted by the drugs is strong and powerful so that it competes with other behavior-controlling factors. For example, drug-DS responding remains intact even when the control of reinforcement schedule is markedly weakened, such as by injecting drugs in toxic doses. Also when behavior itself is severly depressed, the discrimination process may still remain intact. To illustrate, when a high dose of haloperidol was injected to depress response rate to 30% of normal, no deterioration was seen in the animal's ability to select appropriate responses in order to discriminate a narcotic from saline (Gianutsos and Lal, 1975; Colpaert et al., 1975a).

Whereas the relevance of the stimulus continuity can be studied quite easily in the case of external stimuli, drug produced cues are much more difficult to handle in this respect. Drug stimuli can not be switched on or off like external stimuli. However, it may be feasible in the future to approximate the situation by a continuous or discontinuous injections of drugs through intravenous or intraventricular cannula. Also, specific antagonists may be used to abruptly terminate the ongoing drug action. The feasibility of this approach was recently demonstrated by Gianutsos and Lal, (1976) who injected naloxone immediately after the morphine treated rats made drug appropriate responses. They showed that the morphine responding animals switched to the saline appropriate responding after the naloxone injection.

E. Similarities with External Stimuli

In psychology it is well established that whereas different stimuli are discriminated, similar stimuli are generalized. Since a similarity or a difference is not an absolute property, some transfer from one stimulus to another is expected to occur. They are usually represented as a generalization gradient. A subject demonstrates stimulus generalization if, after he has learned to respond to one stimulus, he responds to a second stimulus in a similar way and it bears a quantitative and qualitative relationship to the first. Because characteristic stimulus generalization serves as an important criterion for the establishment of discriminations, it has been extensively investigated by psychologists.

The most obvious way in which the intensity of a drug action can be changed is by changing its doses. Through such an approach it has been demonstrated by many workers that there is a reasonable relationship between the intensity of the training drug-stimulus in the terms of the training drug-dose, and the stimulus generalization along the intensity continuum (dose-response relationship).

In contrast, drug-produced stimuli of different modalities, i.e. different drug classes, are not generalized. They are instead discriminated and some of them demonstrate an unprecedented pharmacological specificity in this respect. Illustrations of such generalizations and discriminations are cited throughout this

book and will not be further elaborated here. However, there
is one point that must be made. In the experiments with external
stimuli two types of procedures are used to establish generalization and/or discrimination. In one situation a stimulus is set
up against the absence of that stimulus. In the other situation
two dimensions or two intensities of the same stimulus are
tested. A parallel situation also exists for the drug stimuli. Two
unlike drugs will not generalize and two sufficiently separate
doses of the same drug will not generalize. In addition, whereas
most often discrimination is established between a drug and a
vehicle, discrimination of two doses of the same drug has been
achieved in many cases

III. DRUG DISCRIMINATION LEARNING VARIABLES

A. Subjects

Drugs have been applied as DS in the man, monkey, gerbil,
rat, mouse and pigeon. No significant species difference has
emerged. All of these species of animals discriminate drug
stimuli. Whereas the higher animals such as humans and monkeys can discriminate more than two drugs from vehicle concurrently, this has not yet been demonstrated in lower animals.
It is interesting to note that the drug discrimination in clinical
studies was reported as early as in 1961 (Frazer et al., 1961).

B. Route of Administration

The routes of administration utilized in drug discrimination
include subcutaneous, intraperitoneal, oral, intravenous and
intraventricular. Future developments will undoubtedly involve
localized intracerebral injections. No qualitative difference based
upon the route of administration has been reported. Nevertheless
the onset and intensity of drug action is determined partly by the
route of administration. Also, whereas a systemic injection will
ensure a generalized drug action, a local injection may sometimes
produce only localized effects and therefore may generate only
a peripherally initiated DS.

C. Dose and Time of Injection

The training dose of the drugs has proved to be a major
variable in the drug discrimination studies. A dose can affect the
discrimination in several ways.

Quantitatively, the training dose determines the intensity of
the set point for discriminative detection. The dose-response
curve obtained from the animals trained on a high dose of a drug

will shift to the right of the dose-response curve similarly obtained in the animals trained on a lower dose. If the curves are parallel as often is the case, the ED_{50} for producing DS will accordingly differ, being higher in the former and lower in the latter case. As a result, the sensitivity of the discriminability is shown to vary over a fairly large range of drug activity using the same essay procedure.

The second consequence of dose effect is seen in the studies on the across-drug generalization. A good example is that of the partial narcotic antagonists (Colpaert et al., 1976a; Colpaert and Niemegeers, 1975). Cyclazocine and nalorphine are narcotic antagonists which also possess some agonist properties. The agonist properties are of low potency which usually generates a bell shaped dose-response curve. Suppose that a narcotic antagonist is tested in three groups of animals which are each trained to discriminate the same narcotic agonist from saline, but in which different training doses have been used. The expected results would be as follows.

The partial agonist-antagonist will show perfect generalization with the narcotic agonist in the test animals which received a low training dose of the agonist. However, if the doses of the same agonist-antagonist beyond ED100 are also tested, they will generate a bell shaped curve. In the animals which are trained with an intermediate dose of narcotic agonist, the agonist-antagonist will show only partial generalization so that the bell shaped dose-response is obtained without reaching ED100. Finally, against the high training dose of a narcotic drug the agonist-antagonist will show very little generalization because the narcotic DS produced by this drug does not match with the high set point of narcotic stimulus ensured by the use of a high dose of the narcotic drug used for training. The preceding hypothetical case is described to illustrate the relevance of the training dose used in the stimulus-generalization experiments in which the generalization even quantitatively depends upon the drug dose used for training, inspite of the fact that the very same training drug is employed.

A third implication of dose effect is found in the differential pharmacological actions produced with different doses of the same drug. This point can be illustrated with the differential DS properties of the low and the high doses of amphetamine (Colpaert et al., 1976a) or morphine (Holtzman, personal communication). Amphetamine produces primarily a peripheral action at very low doses which are essentially devoid of central effects. Consequently rats trained to discriminate a low dose (0.16 mg/kg, d, l amphetamine) generalize the DS with the peripheral action of hydroxyamphetamine. Here low doses of hydroxyamphetamine generalize with amphetamine and high doses of amphetamine generalize with saline. However, the rats trained at a high (2-5 mg/kg) dose of amphetamine no generalization to hydroxyamphetamine takes place (Roffman and Lal, 1972; Silverman and Ho, 1977). In other words, whereas usually the variation in dose employed for training produces DS differing quantitatively, in many cases, a qualitative difference can be demonstrated when a high and a low training dose of the same drug is used for discrimination study.

A result similar to that of amphetamine was found with morphine. Whereas amphetamine and apomorphine do not generalize with morphine in the rats trained to discriminate a higher dose (10 mg/kg) of morphine (Gianutsos and Lal, 1976), both of these drugs generalize with a low dose (0.3 mg/kg) of morphine.

As the drug dose is a critical variable so is the time of injection which also determines the quantity and quality of the drug effect. Hence, discrimination of a drug from saline at different intervals after administration, constitutes a two-sided variable. One, the intensity of action is different and second, the quality of the action may also be different. It has been shown (Gianutsos and Lal, 1976) that the combination of quantity and quality of drug action which is in effect at the time of responding is the determining factor in defining the stimulus. When they are varied because of variation in the time of injection, different drug stimuli may be produced.

There is a practical application of this variable in conducting drug discrimination experiments. In each experiment as drug dose is important because it co-determines quantitative and qualitative aspects of the DS properties of a drug, so is the time of administration before the discriminative responding is begun. Intensity of drug action varies as a function of time, and different actions of the same drug may be produced by different time-effect relations. Hence, requiring an animal to discriminate a drug from saline at different intervals after its administration will pose a problem of varying intensity of drug action, but also one of varying quality of drug actions based upon which the animal is to execute discrimination. These considerations will limit the interpretability of successive discrimination trials within single session following a single drug administration and it is best that a single discrimination trial is run after a constant treatment-interval. This caution is important because the stimulus upon which animals tend to base discrimination is not the one present at the relatively long period preceding the trial but, rather, the one present actually during the trial as was shown in the case of narcotics

(Gianutsos and Lal, 1976).

D. Pharmacological Properties

The drugs used thus far in drug discrimination studies belong to many pharmacological classes. They include anesthetics, sedative-hypnotics, anxiolytics, narcotic analgesics, muscarinic and nicotinic cholinergic agonists, cholinergic antagonists, dopamine-receptor agonists, amphetamines, psychotomimetics, marihuana constituents, antidepressants, and neuroleptics. Based upon these examples there emerges no particularly new qualification that is required of the drugs to be discriminated. Any drug, whatever its nature, which produces a perceivable change anywhere in the body is expected to provide a discriminative control over behavior. It was earlier thought that only CNS active drugs can be discriminated (Overton, 1971). However, recent data with isopropamide (Colpaert et al., 1975b) and hydroxyamphetamine (Colpaert et al., 1976b) present exceptions to the rule. Therefore, activity directly in the CNS is not a prerequisite for discrimination.

The drugs of different pharmacological classes differ with respect to the specificity and inclusiveness of the DS they produce. Within the same class, drugs may also differ between one another, and these differences should be considered in the selection of the training drug of the study of the DS properties of a given class of drugs. For example, fentanyl, as compared to morphine, produces much less behaviorally toxic effects at the doses required to induce a distinct and specific DS. As behavioral toxicity constitutes a factor with disrupting influence on learning and performance, it can be predicted that narcotic discrimination will be acquired more effectively with fentanyl than with morphine. In addition, there may exist other differences between the DS properties of different drugs within the same pharmacological class. Obviously, more research is needed to establish as to which drug produces the DS which are most representative of that class.

E. Sources of Stimuli

There are three types of discrimination currently applied in the drug-discrimination experiments. The most often used discrimination is the drug verses saline which has been found very useful for defining specific DS associated with any drug class to establish pharmacological specificity. The second type is discrimination between two doses of the same drug. This discrimination can provide information on quantitative and qualitative aspects of the DS produced by different drug doses. The third

type involves discrimination between two drugs. This type is
particularly useful to obtain information on differences in pharmacological properties of two drugs belonging to the same class.
For example, many neuroleptics are also anticholinergics. If an
animal can discriminate between two neuroleptics such as
haloperidol and clozapine, one of which is devoid of anticholinergic
properties the discrimination between the two may be based upon
the presence or absence of this extraneous property. However,
there has been very little work done on drug-drug discrimination
to precisely evaluate its usefulness in research.

In addition to the above, one can conceive of several other
discrimination strategies which can be used for specific pur-
poses. They usually involve drug combinations at different doses.
More than two DS may also be used. Generally the availability
of the number and complexity of possible combinations is virtually unlimited.

IV. DISCRIMINATIVE STIMULI AND OTHER PHARMACOLOGI-CAL ACTIONS

There can be no doubt that the DS properties of a drug are
based upon certain physiological changes produced by it. However, little is known of these physiological changes. There are
large numbers of known and probably unknown actions of any
drug. This variation complicates the analysis of the physiological
actions that may be the basis of a drug DS. The present approach
to this problem has been to compare and contrast the DS of a
drug with other concurrently occuring pharmacological actions of
the same durg.

A. Rate of Operant Responding

Most procedures for measuring drug discrimination include
a simultaneous measure of the effect of drugs on the rate of
operant behavior. With the drugs studied thus far the changes
in the rate of responding as induced by a particular dose of any
drug is not related to its potency in producing DS. Most drugs
are discriminated at doses that do not affect response rates, and
they do **not** generalize with different drugs even when tested in
doses that affect response rates.

B. Electrophysiological Changes

No systematic study has been reported that relates DS with
EEG changes produced by drugs. Bliss (1974) reviewed previous
literature which compared the EEG effects of the drugs at doses
which produce state dependent learning. Although he found some
relationship in the case of barbiturates and atropine, the doses

employed were several times higher than those needed to establish a DS using the same drugs.

C. Analgesia

Analgesia is a salient-pharmacological property of narcotic drugs. It can be expected that analgesia may be correlated with DS produced by analgesic drugs. However, a recent investigation produced contrary results. The data have been discussed elsewhere in this book (Lal, et al., 1977) and will not be reviewed here. It is sufficient to say that the discrimination of a narcotic stimulus, although correlated with analgesia, was not based upon the perception of analgesia by the subjects.

D. Euphoria and Abuse Potential

Acquisition and continuation of a drug abuse is usually based upon the specific actions of the drug on the CNS. Not enough is known to define this CNS activity precisely. It is said to be some sort of euphoria effect which is described as a feeling of satisfaction or a "high" (for a discussion, see Lal, 1976). According to Eddy et al., 1970, "this mental state is the most powerful of all the factors involved in chronic intoxication with psychotropic drugs, and with certain types of drugs it may be the only factor involved even in most intense craving and perpetuation of compulsive abuse". The most basic requirement for a drug to be considered as euphorogenic or dysphorogenic is that this drug must cause a CNS action which can be clearly perceived subjectively. It is reasonable to assume that if the CNS effects of a drug can not reach the threshold of perception, that they will not be regarded as euphorogenic or dysphorogenic. Once the CNS effect of a drug is readily perceived, i.e. discriminated, and if that effect generalizes to the euphoric effect of a training drug which is abused, in all likelihood, the new drug will possess high abuse potential. On the other hand, if the perceived (or discriminated) stimuli generalize to those produced by dysphoric training drugs, the test drug would not be expected to be abused. Also if the drug action can not be perceived as shown by a failure to form a DS, this drug is not likely to be abused. According to Frazer et al., (1961), "if one were to select, on the basis of single doses, the most important single subjective response identifying a drug as being subject to morphine-like abuse property this measure would be whether the former opiate addicts identify this drug as an opiate." Therefore, generalization to saline may predict non-abusability and generalization to a drug having a proven abuse potential would predict abuse potential of that drug class.

It should be stated that there are drug abuses which are unrelated to the subjective effects of drugs. Instead such drugs are abused for other reasons such as to prevent insomnia or withdrawal, when the drugs are not prescribed by a physician. These abuse types, of course, will not be associated with the drug DS as the basic reason for their abuse is not to experience euphoria.

E. State Dependent Learning

Relationship between the DS produced by drugs and state dependent learning has been reviewed in another chapter of this book by Colpaert and will not be discussed here. The readers are directed to refer to Colpaert (1977).

V. RESEARCH APPLICATIONS

The research applications of drug induced DS are numerous. Some of them are illustrated below but this is not intended to be an exhaustive list. As the research in this field is progressing rapidly new applications are continuously becoming apparent.

A. Psychology

1. Stimulus Control

Many, if not all, behavioral emmissions of animals and humans are controlled by stimuli, some of which are known and others are yet unidentified. No study of behavior can be undertaken without a careful consideration of stimulus control. Therefore, investigations of stimulus control on behavior occupies a central position in psychological research. Drug-induced stimuli provide a novel tool to study the stimulus control. Before the demonstration of the stimulus properties of specific drugs, existence of chemical stimuli were unknown in the field of psychology. At present it is not known if drug stimuli and the external stimuli follow similar rules. Therefore a new field of research is open for research to answer many questions arising out of the use of chemical stimuli.

2. Experimental Measure of Subjective Effects

Presently, research on cognitive and subjective **perceptions** is limited to experiments with human subjects. This is because there has been complete lack of animal models to study those paradigms. Learning of discriminable stimuli produced by drugs provide a new hope that subjectively perceived alterations in the 'mind' of animals can be measured. DS produced by drugs are related to their subjectively perceived effects in many cases. Therefore, their study will provide information on mechanisms by which the subjective effects are produced and perceived.

Hitherto it was impossible to measure euphoric and dysphoric actions of drugs and other environmental situations because of the lack in measurement technology. They may now be measured by experimentally manipulating the drug-induced euphoria and dysphoria as DS.

3. Interoceptive Stimuli

There has been a long controversy over the existence and characterizations of interoceptive stimuli which are discriminable. DS produced by drugs offer a new tool to investigate the existence of and characterization of interoceptive stimuli in animals. The availability of this tool should provide answers to many questions that have been raised in this area.

B. Disease Models

The learning of internally produced discriminable stimuli is not limited to drugs alone. It is quite conceivable that other changes due to disease states can also be perceived and demonstrated by using the tool of drug discrimination. This is a new approach to bioassay a disease state which can be best described through illustrations of possible applications. It is hoped that these applications will be experimentally tested in future to establish their feasibility.

A drug may be selected to produce hyperthermia and be shown to be discriminated by a laboratory animal. If it is established that the drug discrimination was based upon the hyperthermia produced by this drug, this would provide a paradigm in which a disease state (fever) can be behaviorally discriminated. Whenever, there is a disease condition which either produces hyperthermia or relives an already elevated body temperature it could be behaviorally detected by the trained animals. Fever production would be generalized to the training drug and fever elimination would be discriminated from it. This is one illustration of how a disease state such as fever can be bioassayed with drug discrimination technology.

If we find ways to produce different diseases in experimental animals and have no way of characterizing those diseases without sacrificing the animals, the drug discrimination procedure may be found handy. For example, there is no experimental method to directly detect headache in experimental animals. Also, in normal animals aspirin-saline discrimination is difficult. But if one can train animals to discriminate aspirin in the presence of and not in the absence of a potential headache and since we know that aspirin is an effective drug against headache, we can devise an experimental procedure capable of detecting headache in an animal. Here discrimination of aspirin will be employed to bioassay headache. Similar procedures can be developed to bioassay several other disease conditions. As long as there is a drug known to provide relief from a symptom which is specific of that disease, the presence or absence of this disease can be determined by the use of drug discrimination. It is very likely that this approach can be applied to bioassay anorexia, constipation, pain, inflamation, hypertension, depression, anxiety and even paranoid schizophrenia. We certainly do not mean that the diseases will be real but we are talking about their animal models. Some of these ideas have already been tried. Weissman (1976) found that normal animals do not readily discriminate action of aspirin. However, they readily learned to discriminate aspirin in the presence of chronic pain. Similarily it was found that specific neuroleptics such as haloperidol are very difficult to discriminate because they do not produce subjective effects. However, animals treated with amphetamine rapidly learn to discriminate small doses of haloperidol. We are currently investigating discrimination of antidepressant drugs in reserpine treated animals and of clonidine in genetically hypertensive rats, in order to establish experimental models of depression and hypertension as they are applicable to drug screening.

C. Pharmacology

Drug-induced DS can be a handy tool in pharmacological research. The stimulus itself is a specific pharmacological action of a drug. This action is specific to a drug and its class. In that aspect, the DS follows pharmacological rules of dose-dependency and time dependency. Because of these characteristics, the DS can be applied to verify the pharmacological characterization of a known drug and predict the pharmacology of new drugs. In some instances it can be used for pharmacological characterization which has not been possible through other procedures.

1. Drug Classification

As has been described in an earlier section, the DS produced by drugs can be used to classify new drugs into various pharmacological categories or classes as well as to establish their mechanism of action. Several illustrations of this use have been described throughout this book. They suggest that there are sufficient data now available to demonstrate that DS can be reliably used for predicting drug classification particularly in case of narcotic analgesics, sedatives, psychotomimetics, nicotinics, muscarinics, dopamine agonists, and amphetamines. Others have not been yet extensively investigated.

2. Mechanism of Drug Action

A critical question in pharmacology is to establish the biochemical mechanisms underlying each of the specific drug actions. Because the drug produced DS is a specific action that can be reliably measured, it is a potentially good tool to establish drug mechanisms. It is particularlly useful where the objective is to determine the mechanisms underlying the elicitation of subjective feelings by the drug because no other procedure lends itself to the study of this aspect of drug actions in animals. The biochemical mechanism underlying various actions of the same drug are not necessarily the same. For example, whereas the drugs which alter brain neurotransmitters are known to modify the analgesic actions of narcotics, no such alteration is produced in the DS produced by narcotics (Gianutsos and Lal, 1976; Colpaert, 1976; Lal **et al.**, 1977). This is the first concrete instance in which subjectively perceived actions of drugs are mechanistically separated from the other actions of the same drug.

3. New Drug Property

Induction of DS produced by a drug is a new addition to the list of various actions of drugs. In as much as it is related to euphoria or dysphoria produced by the drugs, it lends itself to their quantitative and qualitative characterization in the laboratory animals. Full potential of this property of drugs has yet to be realized.

D. Drug Development

1. Screening of New Drugs

An important application of drug induced DS is in the field of drug development. The DS are usually produced by very low doses of the CNS action of drugs and they are associated with very specific drug actions. For example, the ED50 values for the narcotics in producing DS are markedly lower than those produced by measuring analgesia in the same animals (Colpaert et al., 1976c; Lal, et al., 1977; Niemegeers, et al., 1976; Miksic & Lal, 1977). The discrimination procedure has been proven useful for screening analgesics, narcotic-antagonists, CNS stimulants, hypnotics, and anxiolytics. For example, in case of narcotic antagonists doses as low as 0.1 mg/kg are readily detected (Gianutsos and Lal, 1976). Potential for screening neuroleptics, antidepressants, antihypertensives, antidiarrheals, and anorexants by this method is currently being investigated.

2. Screening for Specific Actions

An area in which DS techniques may be particularly valuable is to provide a screening procedure in which a drug can be evaluated for specific therapeutic action without interference from side effects. To illustrate, animals may be trained to discriminate an anxiolytic drug against a mildly depressant drug to use them for testing new anxiolytics with no sedative properties. In another situation an undesirable action of a drug may be blocked prior to its use as a training drug. As long as an antidote of a side effect is available it can be combined with a drug to be discriminated so that the drug actions in the presence of antidoted side effect is used as a training drug and new drugs can be sought that generalize to that action. Need for such a type of differentiation among drugs at the time of screening exist in a wide variety of pharmacological areas. Narcotic antagonists without agonists properties, neuroleptics without sedation and extrapyramidal side effects, anticonvulsants without sedation, antihistaminics without sedation, anorexants without CNS stimulation, and antidepressants without autonomic side effects are only a few examples of the CNS drugs which could be screened in drug discrimination tests.

3. Development of New Antagonists

New chemicals can be sought to antagonize stimuli produced by specific drugs. For example, whereas no other drug is known to block narcotic stimuli, narcotic antagonists do that very well. Comparable antagonists which are specific to barbiturates, amphetamines, cocain and alcohol are not yet available. The discrimination procedure can be employed to discover and evaluate such antagonists. Whereas other procedures can be used to detect antagonists at biochemical levels or physiological levels, the discrimination technique specifically determines if the potential antagonist is useful to block 'subjective' effects of the psychoactive drugs. Drug discrimination procedure may be critical where other procedures are not available. Where other procedures are available, the discrimination techniques provide more economical alternatives, as once trained, the same animals are used repeatedly throughout their life span.

4. Animal Models

On several important grounds, human subjects can not be used for drug screening. Therefore we must depend upon laboratory animals to evaluate new chemicals thought to be effective against any one of the vast number of diseases affecting mankind. A limiting factor is that animal models of certain human diseases are hard to find. DS produced by drugs provide an approach which could by utilized to approximate several human disease conditions in the animals for the purpose of drug screening and research. This is particularly valuable in situations where other animal models are not available. For example, there is no good model of headache to screen antiheadache drugs. Generalization with aspirin as described before offers a new approach. Similarly, generalization with clonidine in genetically hypertensive animals may serve as a procedure of screen antihypertensive drugs.

5. Reminder Drug

If a drug is found to be potent eliciter of DS but lacking other pharmacological action, it can be useful as a reminder drug (Weissman, 1976). For example such a drug may be dispensed with a vitamin pill or a birth control pill. For a busy individual a need to remember if these pills were taken on a particular day or not will be minimized. One would know the answer because of the presence or absence of the subjective feeling produced by the reminder drug. Such a drug also provides a unique tool for a study of subjectively perceived mood alterations in the absence of other pharmacological actions.

6. Warning Stimuli

DS induced by drugs may be employed in training of the patients to subjectively perceive physiological signals often produced prior to the onset of certain symptoms. For example, if it is true that convulsive drugs can produce DS at subconvulsive doses, those DS may generalize to the physiological effects of pre-convulsive state. If so, sub-convulsive doses of selected drugs may be used to train patients to clearly discriminate stimuli usually produced prior to an onset of an epileptic seizure. Thereafter, whenever those stimuli become manifested the patient may be treated to block the oncoming seizure.

VI. CONCLUSION

Discriminative stimuli are physical or biological events which reliably control behavior that occurs in their presence or immediately following them. A response is reinforced in the presence of a discriminative stimulus. In its absence that particular response is not reinforced but a different one may be reinforced. Until recently physical events occurring only in the environment of an organism were considered as potential stimuli. However, with the advances in psychopharmacology research, it has become clear that many drug actions can serve as discriminative stimuli. Animals can be trained to emit one of two different responses depending upon whether they have received a drug or a drug vehicle. During training, a drug is administered to the experimental subjects on certain days and drug-appropriate but not vehicle-appropriate responses are reinforced. On randomly alternating days the vehicle is injected and only vehicle-appropriate responses are reinforced. The subjects thus trained, are tested for drug discrimination by treating them with a test drug and observing them to select a drug-appropriate response in the absence of any other cue (no reinforcement is provided on test trials). Well trained animals reliably select a drug-appropriate response when injected with the training drug and a vehicle appropriate response when injected with saline.

Interest in drug-discrimination learning has been steadily increasing for the last few years. Based upon the review of current literature on the discriminative properties of drugs the following characteristics of drug stimuli become apparent.

    A. Classes of drugs which have been shown to produce discriminative stimuli include anesthetics, sedative-hypnotics, anxiolytics, narcotic analgesics, muscarinic and nicotinic cholinergic agonists, cholinergic antagonists, dopamine-receptor agonists, amphetamines, psychotomimetics, marihuana constituents, antidepressants, and neuroleptics.

    B. Discriminative stimuli produced by most drugs are characteristic of their drug class. Similar to their generalization of physical stimuli, animals can readily learn drug-discriminations which generalize to all of the drugs in the same pharmacological class but to none of the others.

    C. Discriminative stimuli are very specific actions of drugs which are produced at dose levels that do not markedly affect behavioral rates. Drug stimuli are antagonized only by specific antagonists.

    D. Discrimination can be formed to a specific action of a drug where other actions of the same drug may be ignored.

    E. Drug induced stimuli are distinct sensations which are

unlike the sensations produced by usual sensory stimuli.

F. Certain drugs can produce two distinct stimuli based upon the dose used for discrimination training.

G. In conventional experiments tolerance to the discriminative stimuli produced by drugs is not seen. However, in case of narcotic analgesics when the drugs are injected in increasing doses without permitting the subjects to practice discriminative responding, some tolerance has been demonstrated.

H. The stimulus control of behavior as exerted by drug stimuli usually follows the same rules of learning as have been established by psychologists working with physical stimuli of external origin.

I. Drug stimuli can be discriminated by various species of laboratory animals and also by human subjects.

The research applications of drug induced discriminative stimuli are many. These stimuli provide a new dimension in stimulus control where stimuli originating from within the body can be investigated. They also provide experimental measures of what may prove to be perception of the subjective feelings. Development of specific antagonists of the subjectively perceived drug actions becomes possible. The drug stimuli provide a new tool to investigate mechanisms of drug actions that are subjectively perceived. Because of their high specificity discriminative stimuli can be used to pharmacologically identify and classify new drugs. Also, an animal can be trained to perceive discriminative stimulus produced only by a desirable drug action by administering the training drug in combination with antidotes of undesirable side effects. Discriminative responding in the animals thus trained can then be employed to screen new drugs which generalize with the desirable actions of the prototype and not possess undesirable side effects. For example, new drugs may be screened for anxiolytic property without sedation or for neuroleptic action that is exerted without producing neurological side effects. By employing drugs whose actions can be detected only in the presence of a disease state, the discriminative stimuli may provide a measure of the disease state itself such as headache in animals who otherwise can not report headache. For example, in normal animals, stimulus produced by aspirin is hardly detectable. However, in the presence of arthritis the aspirin stimulus is very intense. Therefore, a test condition in which aspirin serves as the discriminative stimulus is likely to indicate a painful state. Because drugs are usually abused for their pleasure producing actions which are only subjectively perceived, the identification

of drug stimuli can assist in identifying new drugs with abuse
potential. Drugs that do not produce discriminable stimuli can be
considered to lack abuse potential. Drugs which produce those
stimuli can be further tested, by other methods, if their stimuli
are pleasure producing, neutral, aversive, and/or resemble
those of established drugs of abuse. Drugs with only pleasure
producing stimuli and/or the stimuli resembling those of other
drugs of abuse possess potential for abuse.

VII. REFERENCES

Barry, H. III: Classification of drugs according to their discriminable effects in rats. Fed. Proc. 33: 1814-1824, 1974.

Bliss, D.K.: Theoretical explanations of drug-dissociated behaviors. Fed. Proc. 33: 1787-1796, 1974.

Colpaert, F.: Narcotic cue and narcotic state. Life Sci., 1976, in press

Colpaert, F.C., Lal, H., Niemegeers, C.J.E. and Janssen, P.A.J.: Investigations on drug produced and subjectively experienced discriminative stimuli. I. The fentanyl cue, a tool to investigate subjectively experienced narcotic drug actions. Life Sci. 16: 705-716, 1975a.

Colpaert, F.C., Niemegeers, C.J.E. and Janssen, P.A.J.: Differential response control by isopropamide: a peripherally induced discriminative cue. Europ. J. Pharmacol. 34: 381-384, 1975b.

Colpaert, F.C., Niemegeers, C.J.E. and Janssen, P.A.J.: On the ability of narcotic antagonists to produce the narcotic cue. J. Pharmacol. Exp. Therp. 197: 180-187, 1976a.

Colpaert, F.C., Kuyps, J.J., Niemegeers, C.J.E. and Janssen, P.A.J.: Discriminative stimulus properties of a low dl-amphetamine dose. Archs, Int. Pharmacodyn. Ther., 1976b, in press.

Colpaert, F.C., Kuyps, J.J., Niemegeers, C.J.E. and Janssen, P.A.J.: Discriminative stimulus properties of fentanyl and morphine: tolerance and dependence. Pharmacol. Biochem. Behav., 1976c, in press.

Colpaert, F.C. and Niemegeers, C.J.E.: Narcotic cuing properties of narcotic agonist and antagonist drugs. Exp. Brain Res. 23: 41, 1975.

Colpaert, F.C.: Drug-produced cues and states: Some theoretical and methodological inferences. In Research Applications of Drug-Induced Discriminable Stimuli, ed. H. Lal, Raven Press, New York, 1977, in press.

Eddy, N.B., Hallach, H., Isabell, H. and Seevers, M.H.: Drug dependence: its significance and characteristics. In Drug Abuse, Data and Debate, ed. P.H. Blaeky, Thomas, Springfield, 1970.

Frazer, H.F., Van Horn, G.D., Martin, W.R., Wolback, A.B. and Isabell, H.: Methods for evaluating addiction liability. (A) Attitude of opiate addicts towards opiate-like drug, (B) A short-term direct addiction test. J. Pharmacol. Exp. Therap. 133: 371-387, 1961.

Gianutsos, G. and Lal, H.: Effect of loperamide, haloperidol and methadone in rats trained to discriminate morphine from saline. Psychopharmacol. 41: 267-270, 1975.

Gianutsos, G. and Lal, H.: Selective interaction of drugs with a discriminable stimulus associated with narcotic action. Life Sci. 19: 91-98, 1976.

Lal, H.: Facts and falacies of addiction liability and abuse potential. In Synthetic Antidiarrheal Drugs. eds. W. Van Bever and H. Lal, Marcel Dekker, Inc., New York, pp. 235-251, 1976.

Lal, H., Miksic, S. and Smith, N.: Naloxone antagonism of conditioned hyperthermia: An evidence for release of endogenous opioid. Life Sci. 18: 971-976, 1976.

Lal, H., Gianutsos, G. and Miksic, S.: Discriminable stimuli produced by narcotic analgesics. In Research Applications of Drug-Induced Discriminable Stimuli, ed. H. Lal, Raven Press, New York, 1977, in press.

Miksic, S., Smith, N., Numan, R. and Lal, H.: Acquisition and extinction of a conditioned hyperthermic response to a tone paired with morphine. Neuropsychobiol. 1: 277-283, 1975.

Miksic, S. and Lal, H.: Tolerance to morphine produced discriminative stimuli and analgesia. Psychopharmacol., 1977, in press.

Niemegeers, C.J.E., Lenaerts, F. and Awouters, F.: In vivo pharmacology of antidiarrheal drugs. In Synthetic Antidiarrheal Drugs. ed. Van Bever and Lal, Marcel Dekker, Inc., pp. 65-114, 1976.

Overton, D.: Discriminative control of behavior by drug states. In Stimulus Properties of Drugs, eds. T. Thompson and R. Pickens, Appleton-Century-Crofts, New York, pp. 87-110, 1971.

Roffman, M. and Lal, H.: Role of brain amines in learning associated with amphetamine state. Psychopharmacol. 25: 195-204, 1972.

Roffman, M. and Lal, H.: Stimulus control of hexobarbitol narcosis and metabolism in mice. J. Pharmacol. Exp. Therap. 191: 358-369, 1974.

Shannon, H.E. and Holtzman, S.G.: Evaluation of the discriminative effects of morphine in the rat. J. Pharmacol. Exp. Therap. 198: 54-65, 1976.

Silverman, P.B. and Ho, B.T.: Characterization of discriminative response control by psychomotor stimulants. In Research Applications of Drug-Induced Discriminable Stimuli, ed. H. Lal, Raven Press, New York, 1977, in press.

Thompson, T. and Pickens, R. (eds.): Stimulus Properties of Drugs, Appelton-Century-Crofts, New York, 1972.

Weissman, A.: Future perspectives in research in drug discrimination, Paper presented at Symposium on "Research Applications of Drug-Induced Discriminable Stimuli, 1976.

SUBJECT INDEX

Abstinence, 64, 66
Abuse potential, 47, 48
Acetylcholine, 40, 114
Acetylmescaline, 145
Acetylsalicylic acid, 41
Adrenergic receptor blocker, 116
Aggressive behaviors
  alcohol, 128
  amphetamine, 128, 132
  apomorphine, 128
  atropine, 124, 125, 128
  THC, 122
Alcohol
  anxiety antagonist, 89
  depressant, 73, 82, 84
  discriminative stimulus, 73-89
  disinhibitory effect, 76, 84
  doses, 79, 80, 81, 82, 83, 87, 88
  ED_{50}, 79
  intraperitoneal, 75-82, 87
  intravenous, 79
  oral, 77
  passivity, 87, 89
  sedative, 73, 84, 85, 88, 89
  time interval, 76, 77, 79-83, 86, 88
  toxicity, 82
Alphaprodine, 32, 34
Amantadine, 112, 113
Amobarbital
  discriminative stimulus, 77
Amphetamine, 9, 18, 40, 41, 57, 65, 99, 101, 105, 107, 108, 109, 110, 111, 112, 113, 114, 115, 116, 128, 130, 132, 145, 147
Amphetamine cue, 74, 76, 85, 87, 107, 108, 116
Analeptics, see Drug Names, 100, 102
Analgesia, 31, 48, 122, 224
Analgesics, see Drug Names

actions, 23, 24
antidiarrheals, 36
antiemetics, 23
discrimination, 23
dose effect, 210
drugs, 47, 100, 121
euphoria, 24
narcotic, 24
peristaltic reflex, 23
relative potency, 34
review, 23
tolerance, 29
Anileridine, 35
Anorexia discrimination, 116
Antagonism, 105, 127, 130, 138, 139, 144, 145, 147, 148, 149, 150, 151
Antibiotics, 121
Anticholinergic, see Drug Names, 145, 148, 150
Anticholinesterase, 148, 150
Anticonvulsant, see Drug Names, 94, 99, 104
Antidepressants, see Drug Names, 121
Antimuscarinics, see Drug Names, 123
Apomorphine, 8, 40, 41, 99, 100, 113, 128
Ataxia, 104
Atropine, 41, 88, 112, 114, 115, 124, 125, 128, 142, 145, 147, 148
Avoidance, see Shock, 122
Azaperone, 41
Barbiturates, see Drug Names, 93, 94, 96, 97, 99, 100, 104, 105
Bemegride
  benzodiazepines, 100, 102, 104, 105
  convulsions, 86

discriminative stimulus 74, 85, 86, 87
passivity, 86
tension, 86
stimulant, 86, 88
Benzodiazepines, see Drug Names, 9, 93, 94, 96, 97, 98, 99, 100, 101, 102, 104, 105, 106
Benzitramide, 32, 33, 35
Blood brain barrier, 109
Bromazepam, 94, 95, 97
Bufotonine, 151
Butorphanol, 32, 48, 51, 52, 61, 63, 66
Butoxylate, 35
Caffeine, 41, 88, 99, 101, 105, 112
Cannabinoids
  and atropine, 124, 125, 128
  and pentobarbital, 124, 125, 128
  and phencyclidine, 124, 125, 128
  aggression, 122
  antagonist, 130
  asymmetrical generalization, 132
  avoidance behavior, 122, 127
  chronic treatment, 129
  cross tolerance, 122
  crude marihuana extract, 126
  Delta-8-THC, 124-129
  Delta-9-THC, 123-133
  depressant effect, 122
  discriminative stimulus, 121-136
  doses, 124, 125
  duration of effect, 130-132
  ED_{50}, 126, 130, 132, 133
  emotion, 122
  escape behavior, 122
  food intake, 122, 126
  generalization, 132
  gerbils, 124, 125, 127, 130-132
  hashish smoke, 127, 130
  impairment of behavior, 123, 127
  inhaled, 124, 125, 130, 132
  intramuscular, 125, 130, 132
  intraperitoneally, 124, 125, 130, 132
  intravenously, 130, 132
  lever pressing rate, 127
  monkeys, 124, 125, 130-132
  non-generalization, 127-129
  onset of effect, 130-132
  orally, 124, 125, 129, 130, 132
  perceived effects, 122
  pigeons, 124, 125, 130-132
  rats, 124, 125, 130-132
  route of administration, 124, 125, 129, 130, 132
  species sensitivity, 127, 132
  specificity, 132
  stimulant effect, 122
  stimulus generalization, 132
  stimulus specificity, 132
  task effects, 124
  11-OH-Delta-9-THC, 126
  tolerance, 122, 127
  vocalization, 122
  water intake, 122
Carbachol, 100, 103
Catacholamines, 114
Chevril, 124, 125, 127
Chloral hydrate
  discriminative stimulus, 74, 76, 77, 78, 85, 87, 88, 94, 96
  passivity, 87, 88
  sedation, 87, 88
Chordiazepoxide
  antagonism, 99, 100
  anxiety antagonist, 73, 84, 88
  arousal, 89
  comparison, 128, 132
  convulsions, 98
  discriminative stimulus, 73, 76, 77, 78, 79, 85, 86, 88, 93, 95, 96, 99
  doses, 79, 85, 86
  ED_{50}, 79, 85, 86
  intraperitoneal, 79, 86
  narcotic cue, 41
  sedation, 89, 97
  toxicity, 86
Cinanserin, 114, 115, 146, 148, 150
Clonidine, 41
CNS arousal, 109, 116
Cocaine, 41, 99, 101, 105, 109, 110, 111, 113, 114, 115, 116, 128, 145
Codeine, 32, 33, 34, 35
Conflict, 123, 124

INDEX 235

Cue, see also under Specific drug cues
  drug produced, 7
Cyclazocine, 32, 41, 48, 50, 53, 54, 55, 56, 61, 62, 63, 64, 65, 66, 67, 142, 144, 147
Cyclohexamine, 142, 148, 149
Cyproheptadine, 40, 41, 146, 147, 148, 150
Demerol, 35
Depressant, see Drug Names, 122, 123, 127
Desipramine, 41
Dexetimide, 40, 41
Dextromoramide, 32, 33, 35
Dextrorphan, 31, 41
Diazepam, 77, 78, 94, 95, 97, 100, 105, 128, 130
Difenoxine, 33, 35, 36
Dimethoxyamphetamine, 112
Dimethoxymethylamphetamine, 112, 113, 145
Dimethoxyphenylethylamine, 113, 145, 147
Dimethyltryptamine, 128, 151
Diphenoxylate, 32, 33, 35
Discrete trial avoidance, 27, 50
Discriminated responding, 27, 114
Discrimination
  acetylcholine, 10
  acquisition, 25, 50, 108, 209
  alcohol, 73
  analgesia, 31, 33, 34, 38, 39
  analgesic, 23
  antagonism, 40
  apparatus, 25
  applications, 3, 43
  assumption, 10
  asymmetrical, 16
  attention, 209, 210
  benzodiazepines, 93
  clinical applications, 42
  concepts, 5
  control, 44, 107, 111, 116
  criterion, 9
  data evaluation, 12
  data interpretation, 12
  depressants, 73
  differential reinforcement, 209
  dose dependence, 33, 210
  dose response, 31, 210, 215
  drug properties, 207
  drug specificity, 33
  effects, 51, 53, 54, 56, 59, 60, 62, 66
  endorphins, 42
  future perspectives, 207
  generalization, 8, 111, 114, 116, 138
  hypothetical data, 11
  learning, 208, 215
  maze escape, 28
  mechanism, 40, 208, 213
  methodology, 5, 8, 9, 10, 107, 114, 162, 164, 209
  narcotic antagonists, 42, 47, 55, 64
  narcotics, 23
  neurotransmitter, 40, 42
  non-narcotic analgesics, 41, 42
  norepinephrine, 40
  operant responding, 24
  past research, 207
  perception, 208
  procedure, 24, 77
  properties, 47, 48, 59
  reinforcement, 27, 166
  research, 42
  research tool, 207
  review, 2
  sensitivity, 164, 166
  serotonin, 40
  shock avoidance, 27
  specificity, 31, 166, 169, 214
  stimulants, 107
  stimulus, 208
  superimposition, 12
  testing, 26
  theoretical, 5, 7
  tolerance, 29, 31, 39
  training, 12, 25, 26
  training dose, 209, 210
  trials, 26
  vs state dependent training, 5, 16
Disinhibitory
  alcohol, 76, 84
  pentobarbital, 84

Disulfiram, 114, 115
Ditran, 128, 132, 137, 139, 142, 144, 145, 146, 147, 148, 149, 150
Diuretics, see Drug Names, 121
DOPA, 113
Dopamine, 116, 148, 150
Dopamine-B-hydroxylase, 114
Dopamine receptors, 116
Double alternation, 138
Drug effects
  anxiety, 73, 84
  arousal, 84
  ED_{50}, 78
  passivity, 84, 85
  sedation, 84
  tension, 84, 85
Drug sensitivity
  species, 127, 132
Drug stimulus, see Drug Names, also see Discrimination
Dysphoria, 48, 66, 144
Emotionality, 122
Ephedrine, 113
Ethanol, 111, 122, 128
Ethyl carbamate
  discriminative stimulus, 73, 75
Etonitazine, 32, 34
Euphoria, 48, 61, 66, 114
Fenfluramine, 116
Fentanyl, 8, 14, 15, 16, 17, 30, 31, 32, 33, 36, 40, 55, 64, 67
Fluperamide, 35
Flurazepam, 94, 95, 97
Food
  intake, 122
  reinforcement, 49, 74, 75, 76, 77, 78, 79, 80, 82, 85, 86, 87, 88, 124, 126
Glaucoma, 121
Glutethimide, 76, 94, 97
Hallucination, 137, 150
Hallucinogen, 88, 121, 127, 137, 138, 139, 140, 142, 145, 146, 147, 148, 149, 150, 151
Haloperidol, 9, 40, 41, 42, 94, 115, 144, 148, 150
Hashish, 124, 125, 127, 129, 130
Heroin, 32, 34

Hydroxyamphetamine, 112
Hydroxylase inhibitor, 148
Hyperactivity, 116
Hypnotics, see Drug Names, 121, 123
Hypotensive agents, 121
Imipramine, 41, 147, 148
Indole amine, 140, 144
Indomethacin, 41
Inhalation, 130
Iproniazid, 112, 113, 116
Isomethadone, 32, 34
Isoniazid, 100, 102, 105
Isopropamide, 41
Ketamine, 41, 57, 88, 142, 148, 149
Ketocyclazacine, 41, 53, 61, 64
Levallorphan, 41, 53, 61, 63, 128, 129, 130
Levorphanol, 31, 32, 34
Loperamide, 35, 36, 41
Lorazepam, 94, 95, 97
LSD, 41, 111, 112, 128, 132, 137, 139, 140, 141, 142, 144, 147, 148, 149, 150
Meperidine, 32, 34, 73, 75, 77
Mescaline, 41, 57, 65, 100, 101, 111, 112, 114, 128, 137, 139, 142, 144, 145, 146, 147, 149
Methadone, 32, 33, 34, 35
Methiothepin, 144, 148, 150
Methoxyamphetamine, 112, 113
Methylamphetamine, 112
Methylmescaline, 145
Methylphenidate, 109, 110, 113, 114, 115, 116
Methyl tyrosine, 41, 42, 114, 115
Methysergide, 114, 115, 146, 147, 148, 150
Morphine, 18, 29, 31, 32, 33, 34, 35, 36, 37, 38, 39, 40, 42, 49, 50, 51, 53, 60, 64, 65, 67, 100, 129, 130
Nalbuphine, 41, 48, 53, 61, 63, 64
Nalmexone, 32, 51, 63
Nalorphine, 41, 47, 48, 53, 54, 55, 57, 61, 63, 64, 65, 66, 144, 149

Naloxone, 41, 57, 59, 147, 148
Naltrexone, 41
Narcotic antagonist, 47, 48, 51, 52, 53, 55, 59, 61, 65, 67, 127
Narcotic cue, 8
Narcotics, see Drug Names
 analgesics, 7, 47, 57, 67, 128
 antagonists, 40
 discrimination, 7, 39, 88
 tolerance, 39
Neostigmine, 103, 147, 148, 150
Neuroleptics, see Specific Drug Names, 93, 94, 96, 148
Nicotine
 and amphetamine cue, 111, 112
 and benzodiazepines, 100, 103, 104
 and morphine, 41
 autonomic ganglia, 155, 156
 discrimination, 157
 EEG, 155, 156
 habituation, 156, 157
 locomotor activity, 156
Nicotine cue
 brain levels, 170, 171
 central, 175-177
 central nicotine generalization 172-174
 dopamine, 177-180
 intraventricular administration, 170-175
 muscarinic, 176, 177
 nicotine metabolites, 171-174
 nicotinic, 176, 177
 norepinephrine, 177-180
 peripheral, 175-177
 5-hydroxytramine, 177
Nikethamide, 112, 116
Nitrazepam, 94, 95, 97, 100
Norephedrine, 113
Norepinephrine, 40, 114
Nortryptyline, 128
Operant response
 alley, 75
 conflict, 76, 86
 differentiation, 114
 food reinforcement, 26, 28
 lever pressing, 74, 75, 76, 78, 82, 85, 86, 87, 88

procedures, 108, 109, 138
rate, 82
reinforcement, 107, 108, 138
schedule, 108
shock avoidance, 28
swimming, 88
T-maze, 75, 77, 78, 79, 86, 88
three-compartment box, 87
two-choice discrete avoidance, 53
two-compartment box, 79
two-lever food, 125
Oxazepam, 94, 95, 97
Oxilorphan, 41, 53, 54, 55, 61, 63, 65
Oxotremorine, 112
Oxymorphanol, 32
Oxymorphone, 32, 34
p-chlorophenylalanine, 7, 87, 114 115, 148
Para-chloroamphetamine, 40, 41, 147, 150
Para-hydroxyamphetamine, 108, 109, 112
Partial agonists, see Drug Names
Pentazocine, 32, 48, 49, 51, 52, 55, 59, 60, 61, 62, 63, 64, 66, 67, 139, 149
Pentobarbital
 amphetamine, 111
 arousal, 84, 85, 87, 89
 benzodiazapines, 104, 105
 discriminative stimulus, 9, 41, 73-89, 96, 124, 125, 132
 disinhibitory effect, 85
 doses, 79, 80, 81, 82, 83, 85, 86
 ED_{50}, 79, 85, 86
 intraperitoneal, 78, 81, 82, 83
 intravenous, 79
 learning, 127
 oral, 77
 sedative, 73, 84, 85, 88, 89
 THC, 128
 time interval, 76, 77, 79, 81, 82, 83
 tolerance, 122
 toxicity, 86, 94, 97

Pentylenetetrazol, 74, 85, 87, 94, 96, 98, 100, 102, 104, 105
Peripheral activity, 109, 116
Phenacetin, 41
Phenazocine, 32, 34, 35
Phencyclidine, 88, 124, 125, 128, 132, 137, 144, 147, 148, 149, 150
Phenitrone, 128, 130
Phenobarbital, 73, 75, 94, 96, 97, 100, 128, 132
Phenoperidine, 32, 35
Phenoxybenzamine, 114, 115
Phenoxylate, 36
Phentolamine, 114, 115
Phenylbutazone, 41
Phenylethylamine, 112, 113, 116, 140, 147
Physostymine, 41, 57, 100, 103, 146, 148, 150
Picrotoxin, 100, 102, 105, 112, 116, 147
Pilocarpine, 40, 42
Pimozide, 115, 147
Piritramide, 32, 34
Placebo, 138, 139
Profadol, 48, 51, 52, 57, 58, 61
Propiram, 48
Propoxyphene, 32, 33, 34
Propranolol, 40, 87, 113, 115, 147
Psychotomimetic drugs, see Drug Names, 99, 100
Psychomotor stimulant, see Drug Names, 100, 101, 137, 144
Psilocybin, 112, 128, 137, 140, 142, 145, 149
Punishment, 108
Quanternary cocaine, 109
Quipazine, 144, 149
Receptor, 144, 148, 150
Reserpine, 114, 115
Response
  avoidance, 49, 127
  extinction, 108, 110, 139
  generalization, 111, 113
  operant responding, 49
  reinforcement, 74
  reinforcement schedule, 138, 139
  scope, 74, 78, 82, 83, 85, 88, 122, 123, 124, 125, 137
  selection, 14
Rope climbing, 127
Roto-rod, 127
Scopolamine, 48, 57, 65, 128, 142, 144
Sedative, see Drug Names, 123
Sedation
  alcohol, 73, 84, 85, 88, 89
  chlorpromazine, 87
  drug effect, 84
  ethyl carbamate, 73
  pentobarbital, 73, 84, 85, 88, 89
  phenobarbital, 73
Serotonin, 40, 87, 114, 144, 148, 149, 150
Sleep, 122
Spinal reflexes, 48
Spipeperone, 42
Spontaneous activity, 122
State dependent learning, 5, 7
Stimulant response control, see Drug Names, 107, 114, 116
Stimulants, 107, 121, 122, 127
Stimulus
  auditory, 207
  aversive, 59, 213, 214
  categories, 6, 207, 213
  characteristics, 207, 214
  conditional, 209
  continuity, 214
  control, 18, 209
  cue, 208
  discriminability, 208, 215
  eliciting, 208
  external, 208, 212, 214, 215
  function, 209
  generalization, 17, 48, 55, 93, 214
  internal, 212, 214
  mechanism, 208
  reinforcement, 213
  sensory, 211, 212
  strength, 212
  visual, 207
STP, 112, 113

Strychnine, 100, 102, 105, 112, 116, 117
Sulfentanil, 32, 34
Suprofan, 42
Tacrine, 128, 130, 146, 148, 150
Tail-withdrawal
  analgesia, 36, 38
  drug effect, 37
  latency, 39
  tolerance, 36, 37
Taste aversions, 122
Temporal parameter, 130
Tetrabenazine, 147, 148
Thebaine, 42

T-maze, 108, 123, 124, 138
Tolerance, 18, 122, 127, 140
Tolmetin, 42
Transfer, 138, 139, 140, 144, 148, 149, 151
Tremorine, 103
Trimethoxyphenylacetaldehyde, 145
Trimethoxyphenylethylamine, 145
Trimethoxyphenylethanol, 145
Tryptamine, 100, 102, 105, 112
  twitch response, 48
  vocalization, 122
  xylamidine, 147, 148
  yohimbine, 128, 147, 158

DATE DUE			
OCT 3 1 1993			
	MAR 2 9 1994		
OCT 0 4 1993			
APR 0 4 1994			

DEMCO 38-297